Integrated Management of Depression in the Elderly

Edited by

Carolyn Chew-Graham
University of Manchester

Robert Baldwin
Manchester Mental Health and Social Care Trust

Alistair Burns
University of Manchester

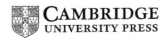
CAMBRIDGE
UNIVERSITY PRESS

CAMBRIDGE UNIVERSITY PRESS
Cambridge, New York, Melbourne, Madrid, Cape Town, Singapore, São Paulo, Delhi

Cambridge University Press
The Edinburgh Building, Cambridge CB2 8RU, UK

Published in the United States of America by Cambridge University Press, New York

www.cambridge.org
Information on this title: www.cambridge.org/9780521689809

First published 2008

Printed in the United Kingdom at the University Press, Cambridge

A catalogue record for this publication is available from the British Library

ISBN 978-0-521-68980-9 paperback

Contents

Contributors   *page* vi

Foreword

by Dan Blazer   xiii

Preface   xv

Acknowledgements   xvi

1   Late-life depression: an introduction   1

2   Management of late-life depression   17

3   Management of late-life depression in primary care: case
     studies UK   33

4   Management of more complicated depression in primary
     care: case studies UK   55

5   Management of late-life depression across primary
     and secondary care: case studies UK   83

6   Management of late-life depression around the world:
     summary of international commentaries   102

7   Resources   114

     Appendix: International commentaries   140

Index   178

Contributors

UK contributors

Dr Harry Allen
Consultant in Old-Age Psychiatry
Manchester Mental Health and Social Care Trust

Professor David Challis
Professor of Community Care Research
Personal Social Services Research Unit
University of Manchester

Dr Mike Cheshire
Consultant in Medicine of the Elderly
Central Manchester and Manchester Children's Hospital Trust

Dr Simon Cocksedge
General Practitioner and Lecturer in General Practice
The Medical School
University of Manchester

Dr Avril Danczak
General Practitioner and GP Tutor and Trainer
Manchester Primary Care Trust

Dr Ceri Dornan
General Practitioner and GP with Special Interest (Mental Health)
Manchester Primary Care Trust

Professor Christopher Dowrick
General Practitioner and Professor of Primary Medical Care
School of Population, Community and Behavioural Sciences
University of Liverpool

Dr Chris Fox
Consultant and Senior Lecturer in Psychiatry
Kent Institute of Medicine and Health Sciences
University of Kent

Dr Jane Hughes
Lecturer in Community Care Research
Personal Social Services Research Unit
University of Manchester

Professor Steve Iliffe
General Practitioner and Professor of Primary Care
Royal Free and University College Medical School
London

Professor Cornelius Katona
Dean
Kent Institute of Medicine and Health Sciences, University of Kent

Ahmed I. Lambat
Manager and Social Work Practice Teacher/Assessor
The Pastoral Centre
Manchester

Professor Helen Lester
General Practitioner and Professor of Primary Care
Primary Care Research Group
School of Community Based Medicine
University of Manchester

Professor Karina Lovell
Professor of Mental Health Nursing
School of Nursing, Midwifery and Social Work
University of Manchester

Dr Sue Martin
Independent Practitioner and Trainer
Liverpool

Dr Michael Morley
Consultant Clinical Psychologist
Manchester Mental Health and Social Care Trust

Dr Elizabeth Murray
General Practitioner and Reader in Primary Care
Royal Free and University College Medical School
London

James Oliver
Substance Abuse Counsellor
Lonsdale Medical Centre
London

Dr Joanne Protheroe
General Practitioner and Clinical Research Fellow
Primary Care Research Group
School of Community Based Medicine
University of Manchester

Helen Pusey
Lecturer in Nursing
School of Nursing, Midwifery and Social Work
University of Manchester

Dr Greta Rait
General Practitioner and Senior Lecturer in Primary Care
Royal Free and University College Medical School
London

Dr Joy Ratcliffe
Consultant in Old-Age Psychiatry
Manchester Mental Health and Social Care Trust

Dr Ruth Thompson
General Practitioner
Robert Darbishire Practice
University of Manchester

Dr Waquas Waheed
Academic Consultant Psychiatrist
Lancashire NHS Trust
and
Honorary Lecturer
University of Manchester

Professor Ken Wilson
Consultant in Old Age Psychiatry
Wirral Community Healthcare NHS Trust

International contributors

Australia

Professor David Ames
Professor of Psychiatry of Old Age
Department of Psychiatry
University of Melbourne

Dr Eleanor Flynn
Senior Lecturer in Medical Education
Faculty of Medicine
University of Melbourne

Bulgaria

Associate Professor Maria Alekxandrova
Associate Professor of Psychiatry
Department of Psychiatry
Medical University, Pleven

Dr Kaloyan Stoychev
Consultant Psychiatrist
Department of Psychiatry
University Hospital, Pleven

Canada

Professor Kenneth Shulman
Lewar Chair in Geriatric Psychiatry
Sunnybrook Health Sciences Centre
University of Toronto

Professor Ross Upshur
Chair in Primary Care Research
University of Toronto

Denmark

Dr Kirsten Abelskov
Old Age Psychiatrist
Psychogeriatric Department
Aarhus University Hospital

Kaj Sparle Christensen
General Practitioner
Institut for Almen Medicin
University of Aarhus

France

Dr Michel Benoit
Psychiatrist
Centre Mémoire de Ressources et de Recherche
Nice

Dr Florence Cabane
General Practitioner
Nice

Professor Philippe H. Robert
Professor of Psychiatry
Centre Mémoire de Ressources et de Recherche
Nice

Dr Geneviève Ruault
Geriatrician
Société Française de Gériatrie et de Gérontologie
Nice

Hong Kong

Professor Helen F. K. Chiu
Chairman and Professor of Psychiatry
Department of Psychiatry
The Chinese University of Hong Kong

Professor D. K. T. Li
Past President
Hong Kong College of Family Physicians

Japan

Dr Syuichi Awata
Director
Division of Neuropsychiatry and Center for Dementia
Sendai City Hospital

Dr Akira Honma
Psychiatrist
Department of Psychiatry
Tokyo Metropolitan Institute of Gerontology

The Netherlands

Dr Marijke Bremmer
Consultant Psychiatrist
Institute for Research in Extramural Medicine
VU University Medical Centre
Amsterdam

Dr Els Licht-Strunk
General Practitioner
Institute for Research in Extramural Medicine
VU University Medical Centre
Amsterdam

Norway

Professor Knut Engedal
Professor of Old-Age Psychiatry
Ullevaal University Hospital
Oslo

Professor Harald Sanaker
Specialist in Family Medicine
Kongsvegen Legesenter
Brummunddal

Romania

Dr Monica Bălan
Primary Care Physician
Oradea

Dr Alexandru Dicker
Senior Consultant in Internal Medicine
Psychiatric Hospital Nucet
Bihor

Dr Nicoleta Tătaru
Senior Consultant Psychiatrist
Forensic Hospital Ştei
Bihor

Spain

Dr Jose Antonio Ferreiro Guri
Specialist in Family and Community Medicine
University of Santiago de Compostela

Professor Raimundo Mateos
Professor of Psychiatry
University of Santiago de Compostela

USA

Professor Tom Campbell
Professor of Family Medicine
Lovejoy Family Medicine Center
University of Rochester
Rochester, NY

Professor Jeff Lyness
Professor of Psychiatry
University of Rochester Medical Center
Rochester, NY

Foreword

To my knowledge there is nothing quite like this book in the English language, perhaps in any language. This is not to say late-life depression has not been the focus of previous books. Felix Post, in 1962, published the results from his clinical follow-up of late-life depression in what I believe was the first text for physicians on the symptoms and course of this common condition written in the twentieth century.[1] I attempted a general overview of the topic twenty years later, summarizing the extant literature and coupling this review with my own experience in treating depressed older adults.[2] The National Institutes of Mental Health in the United States convened a consensus panel a little over a decade later that lead to a detailed literature review and recommendations for clinical investigators, recommendations that have spawned a plethora of research reports over the past decade.[3] There have been many other single-authored and edited textbooks since.

What makes this book different? Is this difference of use to practitioners? Unlike anything written to date, the editors have derived their primary data from the most important source for truly grasping the nature of late life depression and entering the complex task of designing and implementing a treatment plan. That source is the collection of practitioners 'on the ground' working with depressed older adults daily, beginning not with the psychiatrist or psychologist but with the primary care physician/general practitioner. The perspective of clinicians from a variety of disciplines working in concert to manage depressed elders is the real world of old-age psychiatry. Is this approach of value? Absolutely! Academic physicians, and perhaps physicians in general, have become so enamored with evidence from empirical studies of depression that they often overlook the nuances of treating one older adult in her or his unique environment. They retreat to the sterile environment of diagnosis and treatment algorithms and ignore the individual (there is nothing

---

[1] Post F. (1962) *The Significance of Affective Symptoms at Old Age*. London: Oxford University Press.

[2] Blazer D. (1982) *Depression in Late Life*. St Louis, MO: Mosby.

[3] Schneider L., Reynolds C., Lebowitz B., Friedhoff A. (1994) *Diagnosis and Treatment of Depression in Late Life*. Washington, DC: American Psychiatric Press.

wrong with an algorithm as long as it is adapted to the individual patient in the context of that patient's sociocultural environment).

Many texts describe the importance of a collaborative approach to treatment. Yet these descriptions are usually through the eyes of one discipline. The editors of this text provide the reader the views of multiple practitioners reflecting upon the diagnosis and treatment of an individual patient. It is one thing to say that collaboration is important, it is another to actually listen to one's colleagues' unique disciplinary perspectives. Those who read this book must do just that.

A unique contribution of this text for practitioners is the multicultural perspective. This perspective emerges in at least two ways. First the authors describe the diversity of patients who the primary care physician encounters in the United Kingdom. Yet of more interest, they provide in Chapter 6 a cross-cultural reflection upon a case of old-age depression. I found the Appendix with the actual text of the responses from clinicians across the world especially intriguing. Patients do not simply vary across cultures. Clinicians view their patients differently given the cultural background of the clinician though many approaches to therapy are virtually universal. In our current era of reductionistic biological psychiatry, this variation in perspective is often unacknowledged, if not unknown.

Finally, this book is not only useful but fun. How often can that be said about a medical text? Even for the clinician immersed in the daily care of older adults this book is so unique and so relevant that the reader must engage the text. So I welcome the opportunity to provide this foreward, congratulate the editors, and join what I hope will be a large audience of readers.

Dan Blazer MD, PhD
J. P. Gibbons Professor of Psychiatry and Behavioral Sciences
Duke University Medical Center
Durham, North Carolina, USA

Preface

Depression in older people is common, distressing for patients, and is associated with high morbidity and mortality. It is often unrecognized and usually under-treated. Contrary to much professional and public opinion, depression is treatable with both drug and psychological approaches, which lead to significantly improved health and social outcomes for individuals. The book begins with a review of the epidemiology of depression in older people and then a more in-depth analysis of a number of approaches to management, such as self-care, stepped care and collaborative care.

Our experience in managing depression in older people was heightened by our involvement in a trial which evaluated a collaborative care approach to the management of depression in older people in primary care. Arising from that experience, and our clinical exposure, we have focussed the book on a discussion of a number of clinical cases, based on real cases we have encountered, by practising health and social care professionals around the world. Despite a current vogue for emphasizing individual differences, we were impressed at how the presentation and often the management of older people with depression is common across cultures – or at least, the similarities outweigh the differences. However, the latter are sufficient to build up a fascinating picture from an international perspective.

We hope we have succeeded in making the book appealing to a broad range of readers who work with older people, and that the case commentaries, in particular, will appeal to students of the health and social care professions, as well as primary and secondary care professionals and providers in the voluntary sector.

We wish to thank all of our contributors (listed on pages vi–xii) who invested their time, thoughtfulness and expertise in the commentaries. We particularly wish to thank Ken Wilson and Karina Lovell, who were also involved in our trial, and Waquas Waheed for their contributions.

Acknowledgements

We thank our spouses for their support during the preparation of this book. We are indebted to our patients without whom there would have been no inspiration to write. Special thanks go to Barbara Dignan who organized and managed us.

Late-life depression: an introduction

The epidemiology of depression in later life

Professor Ken Wilson, Consultant in Old-Age Psychiatry, Wirral Community Healthcare NHS Trust

There is debate about the prevalence of depression in later life. Some authors argue that the prevalence of depression is substantially less than in younger populations (Regier *et al.* 1993); others, for example Osborn *et al.* (2003), have found an increase with age in the very old in a large community sample. Recent European studies have found prevalence estimates of between 8.8% and 23.6% (Copeland *et al.* 1999). This variability reflects a wide range of issues which include the various definitions used, and in particular, the associated diagnostic instruments.

Strict criteria which have high specificity or are mainly designed for research purposes are likely to identify fewer depressed individuals in population studies when compared to instruments adopting broader definitions of depression. The Diagnostic and Statistical Manual (DSM-IV) has tightly defined criteria, whereas the Geriatric Mental State Examination identifies a broader range of depressive conditions. Consequently, when compared with DSM-IV criteria, the latter identifies cases across a number of different DSM-IV syndromes, provided that the individual presents with depressive symptoms of a severity warranting therapeutic intervention. This instrument also identifies people with adjustment disorder and dysthymia as well as major depressive disorder (Newman *et al.* 1998, Schaub *et al.* 2003). The close relationship between depression, physical illness and dementia also presents problems for epidemiological investigation. A significant minority of the very old may also experience dementia or high levels of physical illness both of which can mask the clinical presentation of depression. Lastly some studies will include institutionalized older people; others will focus on the relatively independent, living in their own homes. These and many other issues will influence the prevalence and incidence rates reported by each study.

Integrated Management of Depression in the Elderly, ed. C. Chew-Graham, R. Baldwin and A. Burns. Published by Cambridge University Press. © Cambridge University Press 2008.

Despite these problems, epidemiological research provides us with a number of important insights and some consistent findings that not only can inform service provision but also have important, more specific clinical implications for both primary and secondary care and social care. Population studies have demonstrated that depression is one of the commonest mental health problems facing older people. Studies have consistently demonstrated that depression (irrespective of how it is defined) is a significant problem for a substantial minority of older people and studies of older people living in residential homes, nursing homes and other institutions tend to report higher prevalence and incidence rates, which probably reflect the higher prevalence rates of physical illness.

Depression in later life ranges in severity and presentation and 'depression' covers a broad spectrum of disorders. Even a few depressive symptoms (not of the severity that warrant treatment) are associated with future development of more severe depressive illness. The early identification and monitoring of these 'sub-syndromal' symptoms is important and has been included within influential clinical guidelines (NICE 2004). Clinical depression may also fluctuate in severity and nature of presentation across many years of illness (Beekman *et al.* 1995) and it is important to remember that major depression is a recurring disorder with the majority of older patients having a recurrence within three years (Reynolds *et al.* 1999). All the research indicates that untreated depression is associated with poor outcome (in naturalistic studies), resulting in prolonged morbidity and increased use of primary and secondary care resources (Pearson *et al.* 1999).

Even though depressed mood remains a core feature of presentation comparative studies of differing age groups indicate that older people may present with differing symptom emphasis. Examples, which are discussed further in the next section, include an increased experience of physical symptoms (Good *et al.* 1987) and an association with cognitive impairment, both potentially causing diagnostic problems and influencing management and prognosis.

A general consensus is developing with regard to potential risk factors for depression in later life. These have been identified through incidence studies which involve following up non-depressed older people and identifying those factors associated with subsequent depression. It is evident that there is a complicated relationship between handicap, defined as 'disadvantage for an individual resulting from ill health compared with what is normal for someone of the same age, sex and background' (World Health Organization 1980), social isolation and pain and subsequent depression (Prince *et al.* 1997). Adverse conditions such as these are more prevalent in poorer populations which may explain the increased incidence of depression in older people from lower socio-economic groups (Wilson *et al.* 1999a).

These and many other studies have provided us with a profile of 'at-risk' populations. Older, physically ill people living in institutions are at particular risk. Likewise, the prevalence of depression in older people recently discharged from acute medical care is higher than found in the majority of community-based studies (Gerson *et al.* 2004). Depression is a particular problem for the bereaved, the lonely and those living alone (Livingston *et al.* 1990). These and other studies have facilitated targeted screening programmes, enabling the identification of depressed older people in high-risk groups.

The evidence consistently demonstrates that depression is under-diagnosed and under-treated in clinical practice (Wilson *et al.* 1999b). Comparative studies have enabled us to explore how the presentation is influenced by age, age-related factors, social adversity and disease and we are able to provide an informed commentary regarding the nature and course of the condition. High-risk populations are easily identified in community settings. The development of easily delivered screening instruments and evidenced-based pathways of care provide the means for early identification and management of older depressed people in both community and secondary care settings. Despite these advances, one of the main problems confronting the older depressed person continues to be the lack of appropriate assessment, diagnosis and management.

The aetiology of depression in later life

Dr Carolyn Chew-Graham, University of Manchester, and Professor Robert Baldwin, Manchester Mental Health and Social Care Trust

The primary care clinician needs to be aware of the factors in a patient's background that constitute a risk for depression (Box 1.1), and life events that may precipitate an episode (Box 1.2). There are also counterbalancing factors that are protective (Box 1.3), particularly social support and security of the environment, which the clinician should explore with the patient. It is the interplay of these factors which determines whether a person develops depression, rather than one particular factor, and thus why some people develop

---

Box 1.1 Risk factors for depression in later life

- Genetic susceptibility
- Gender (being female, although isolated, elderly males are at particular risk of suicide)
- Past history
- Civil status – widows, widowers and divorcees are at particular risk
- Structural brain changes and vascular risk factors
- Personality
- Physical co-morbidity
- Handicap (deafness, poor vision)

Box 1.2 Precipitating factors for depression in later life

Life events
- Bereavement
- Separation
- Acute physical illness
- Hospital admission
- Change of housing
- Financial crisis
- Loss of significant other (including pet)
- Negative interactions with family member

Chronic stress
- Declining health
- Dependence
- Sensory loss
- Problems (e.g. illness) affecting family member
- Socio-economic decline
- Marital difficulties
- Retirement
- Being a carer
- Social isolation

Other
- Drugs (prescribed and non-prescribed)
- Alcohol

Box 1.3 Protective factors in late-life depression

- Social support
- Coping behaviours
- Good nutrition
- Exercise and physical fitness
- Optimal control of co-morbid problems
- Religious affiliation

---

depression even in the absence of an adverse life event, while in others even one or more major life events does not precipitate a depressive illness.

There is no evidence that ageing per se is a major risk factor for depression. It is important that just because a patient is elderly or has suffered a life event such as bereavement that the depression is not considered 'understandable' and thus thought to be untreatable by the clinician (Burroughs *et al.* 2006).

It is vital that the clinician explores all factors in assessing the older patient presenting with depressive symptoms, probing for both indicators of individual susceptibility and adverse life events. The potential for exploring these factors in the over-75 assessment outlined in the GP Contract (Department of Health 1989) and in the primary care consultation is probably underexploited.

Organic factors are more important to consider in older people than in younger adults, and a drug and alcohol history is vital, including what the patient is buying over the counter. Disability due to physical ill-health is strongly associated with depression and thus should be minimized where possible. Positive social and environmental factors may offset the negative effects of adverse life events and are important areas for public health intervention.

Presentation of depression in later life

Dr Carolyn Chew-Graham, University of Manchester, and Professor Robert Baldwin, Manchester Mental Health and Social Care Trust

Core symptoms

People with depression usually present to primary care clinicians who, in order to make a diagnosis of depression, should ideally explore for core and additional symptoms (ICD-10) (World Health Organization 1993) (Boxes 1.4 and 1.5). The DSM-IV (American Psychiatric Association 1994) classification states that in order to distinguish depression from understandable sadness, the symptoms need to be present for more than two weeks, the symptoms must be present for most days, most of the time, and be of an intensity that is definitely not normal for that person.

Clinical presentation of depression in later life

Major depression in older people is essentially the same as at other times of life and it is untrue to say that depressive disorder in older adults cannot be distinguished from normal ageing, although both patients and clinicians experience difficulty with this, and tend to normalize symptoms (Burroughs *et al.* 2006). For the general practitioner (GP), it is important to consider the following:

- When depressed, older people in Western societies complain less often of sadness that their younger contemporaries.
- Hypochondriasis is consistently reported as a symptom more commonly in late-life depression, and older people are more likely to have co-existent physical illness.

Box 1.4 Main features of depressive disorder

Core symptoms
- Depressed mood sustained for at least two weeks
- Loss of interest or pleasure in normal activities
- Decreased energy or increased fatigue

Additional symptoms
- Loss of confidence or self-esteem
- Inappropriate and excessive guilt
- Recurrent thoughts of death, suicidal thoughts or behaviour
- Diminished evidence of ability to think, impaired concentration
- Change in psychomotor activity (inactivity or agitation)
- Sleep disturbance
- Appetite change and weight change

Box 1.5 Diagnosis of depressive disorder

For *mild* depressive episode
- At least two core symptoms
- Additional symptoms to give a total of at least four symptoms

For *moderate* depressive episode
- At least two core symptoms
- Additional symptoms to give a total of at least six symptoms

For *severe* depressive episode
- All three core symptoms
- At least five additional symptoms
- May be presence of psychotic symptoms or stupor

- Subjective memory disturbance may be a prominent symptom and lead to a differential diagnosis of dementia. Anxiety is a common presenting or accompanying symptom.
- Dementia may alter the presentation of depression and the primary care clinicians should be aware that increased confusion or aggressive outbursts in patients with dementia may be due to co-existent depression.

Making the diagnosis of depression in later life

The primary care clinician needs to have an awareness of the possibility of depression in any older person consulting, particularly those with chronic disease where depressive disorder will be more common. The Quality and Outcomes Framework (QOF) of the new General Medical Services (GMS) Contract (BMA and NHS Employers 2006) requires that GPs and practice nurses use two screening questions within the previous 15 months with patients with chronic disease (Box 1.6).

The clinician needs to be aware of cues, both verbal and non-verbal, exhibited by the patient which would raise the possibility of depression.

Some clinicians use validated schedules to assist in the diagnosis of depression with patients where they already have a high index of suspicion, and the Patient Health Questionnaire-9 (PHQ-9) is now included in the Quality and Outcomes Framework (QOF) of the new GMS contract (BMA and NHS Employers, 2006) in England and Wales (see also Chapter 7, pp. 115–117). There is limited evidence of the effectiveness of the validated tools such as the Geriatric Depression Scale (GDS) for screening of elderly populations in primary care, but it may be useful in certain target populations (Box 1.7) and it does have cross-cultural validity (Rait *et al.* 1999).

Box 1.6 Screening questions for depression

'During the past month, have you often been bothered by feeling down, depressed or hopeless?'
'During the past month, have you often been bothered by having little interest or pleasure in doing things?'

A 'yes' to either question is considered a positive test.
A 'no' response to both questions makes depression highly unlikely.

Box 1.7 Suggestions for targeted screening in primary care

- Recent (<3 months) major physical illness or hospital admission
- Chronic illness
- In receipt of high levels of home care
- Recent bereavement
- Socially isolated people
- Those people persistently complaining of loneliness
- Patients complaining of persistent sleep problems

Rating scales

In primary care, time is at a premium, so rating scales are rarely used. They can, however, provide an additional more objective measure of severity and progress, which can inform treatment decisions. For more information about scales used by clinicians see the following section and Chapter 7.

Clinical evaluation

The clinician should cover five areas in the primary care consultation when suspecting depression (Box 1.8).

Box 1.8 Areas to cover in a primary care evaluation of depression

History
- Sensitive exploration of core and additional symptoms
- Identification of triggers
- Previous history of depression
- Recent bereavement
- Maintaining factors – drugs, alcohol
- List of medications (including benzodiazepines and self-medication)
- Substantiating the history by talking with the a carer or family member (with the patient's consent) can help to clarify aspects of the history

Mental state assessment
- Evidence of psychotic symptoms
- Thoughts of self-harm
- Use of Mini-Mental State Examination (MMSE) where cognitive impairment seems a problem (see also Chapter 7).

Risk assessment
- Thoughts of self-harm
- Plans
- What prevents the patient acting on thoughts or plans

Focussed physical examination
- Focussed neurological examination
- Blood pressure and pulse
- May help identify contraindications to certain classes of antidepressants

Appropriate investigations
In primary care, blood tests including full blood count, biochemistry (including calcium), glucose, liver and thyroid function, haematinics (B_{12} and folate, in particular).

In summary, a comprehensive assessment of depressive disorder in an older person includes taking a history, performing a focussed physical examination, assessing mental state and risk, and arranging relevant blood tests. It should be remembered that those most at risk of suicide are isolated men, aged over 80 years, and those with chronic physical conditions or who use alcohol to excess. A previous history of self-harm or a clinical picture of severe depression also increases risk. Most older people who succeed in killing themselves have consulted a primary care doctor in the month prior to suicide. Whilst clinicians are perhaps more aware of the risks of suicide and the need to carry out a risk assessment, it is sometimes forgotten that older people may harm themselves through self-neglect, and the clinician should be aware of the risk of a patient becoming physically compromised through dietary self-neglect as a result of a depressive illness.

Depression in older people from different ethnic groups

Dr Waquas Waheed, Academic Consultant Psychiatrist, Lancashire NHS Trust and Honorary Lecturer, University of Manchester

Background

The 2001 Census indicated that 7.9% of the population in the UK are of ethnic minority origin. The first post-war migrants to arrive were from the Caribbean, shortly after the Second World War and during the 1950s. Later immigrants from India and Pakistan arrived mainly during the 1960s and Bangladeshi people came to Britain during the 1980s. These groups have a younger age structure than the White population, reflecting past immigration and fertility patterns. Progressive ageing of the minority ethnic population is anticipated in the future, as these groups are fast approaching retirement age, but changes will depend on mortality rates and future net migration (United Kingdom National Census 2001).

The concept of multiple jeopardy postulates that ethnic elders, by virtue of age, socio-economic difficulties and minority status, are at greater risk of illness, thus in greater need of health services (Norman 1985, Rait *et al.* 1996). There is a paucity of research on mental health, access and use of mental health services, health providers' understandings of explanatory models and the need for culturally sensitive services for ethnic elders in the UK.

Prevalence and risk factors for depression

The community prevalence of depression in South Asian elderly people may approach 20% (Bhatnagar and Frank 1997) and is 13–19% in Black people from Africa and the Caribbean (McCracken *et al.* 1997). Similar high levels of symptoms of anxiety and depression and low levels of life satisfaction in both Somali and Bengali elderly people have been reported from inner-city London. These Bengali elderly people compare unfavourably with previous studies among the general population in other parts of Britain, including the under-privileged (Silveira and Ebrahim 1998).

Prevalence of depression, self-harm and suicide is also higher amongst ethnic minority adults of working age, particularly women. Psychosocial issues in the realms of poor housing, racial discrimination, low literacy, lack of English language skills, isolation, lack of support and difficulties in marital and family relationships are the reasons cited for this elevated prevalence in ethnic minorities. This is further compounded by different traditional or religious expectations and beliefs about marriage, divorce, widowhood and family honour (Husain *et al.* 1997, Chew-Graham *et al.* 2002, Khan and Waheed 2006).

Age-related factors commonly observed in the lives of older people from ethnic minorities further contribute to this high prevalence. A majority of people aged over 65 are said to suffer from a chronic medical condition that impairs their ability to function and makes them more vulnerable to depression (Unützer *et al.* 1999). This gains further importance due to the fact that prevalence of diabetes, heart disease and other chronic medical conditions is much higher in ethnic elders (Bhopal *et al.* 2002). It has been observed that higher psychological morbidity occurred amongst bereaved Caribbean individuals, with family doctors cited as a source of support for three-quarters of these respondents, who therefore may need to focus on the culture specific needs of these communities (Koffman *et al.* 2005).

This higher prevalence must be seen in the context that Asian and Black elders are more likely to consult their GP than White elders (Blakemore 1982, Murray and Williams 1986) yet they are referred less to secondary care health and social services, particularly psychiatric services (Shah and Dighe-Deo 1997). Several reasons have been suggested for the lack of utilization of psychiatric services. Interpreting symptoms as a spiritual problem (Kleinman 1987) or a physical illness (Odell *et al.* 1997); reluctance of ethnic elders to accept referral to secondary mental health services (Shah *et al.* 1998); and perceptions by Black people of racism in health workers (Hutchinson and Gilvarry 1998) are cited as the main reasons.

The majority of older people do not view depression as a mental illness. Ethnic elders particularly do not see psychiatric services as appropriate and believe they are primarily for psychosis and violence. These views are amenable to change. Doctors should be explicit that services include people with depression (Marwaha and Livingston 2002).

Symptoms and course of depression

It may be that medical professionals are less able to recognize the presentation of psychological distress by people from other cultures. During qualitative interviews with diverse ethnic elders, depression was often viewed as an illness arising from adverse personal and social circumstances that accrue in old age. White British and Black Caribbean participants defined depression in terms of low mood and hopelessness; South Asian and Black Caribbean participants frequently defined depression in terms of worry (Lawrence *et al.* 2006).

People across cultures often present with culturally specific idioms of distress. South Asians often describe their distress using 'sinking heart' or 'gas in abdomen' (*gola*) as a symptom of distress. This often misguides the clinicians and they tend to overlook the psychological distress and focus on solely on physical aspect of the presentation (Krause 1989).

Patients particularly from ethnic minorities have misconceptions about depression. The following are examples of common beliefs held:

- Antidepressants are addictive.
- Antidepressants treat the symptoms, not the causes, of depression.
- I should be able to cope with depression on my own.
- I can't be depressed – I've no reason to be.
- Being depressed is a weakness – it's not a proper illness.
- All antidepressants are the same.
- My depression will get better by itself.

To improve care for depressed ethnic elders, health-care providers must integrate knowledge of ethnicity and culture into their practice, which will help in dispelling these misconceptions. Therefore, it is useful to elicit ethnic elders' explanatory models and beliefs about their depression which will not only help in better understanding between the two parties but will help in negotiating treatment and setting therapy goals. Cultural presentation and conceptualization of depression combined with the patients' expectations regarding treatment and health services has a huge impact on how they seek, receive and adhere to the treatment plans. A culturally sensitive assessment is pivotal for providing safe, appropriate, and quality care to this often misunderstood and under-served population.

Another important factor is that symptoms of depression in ethnic minorities tend to persist for longer periods and follow a chronic course (Husain *et al.* 1997). The main reason for this may be lack of treatment-seeking, treatment provision and/or adherence in this group. This leads to non-resolution of symptoms; thus incidence may be the same but prevalence becomes higher. Depression in older adults is also more likely to follow a chronic course compared with working-age adults irrespective of their ethnicity. The probable reasons for these large discrepancies between prevalence, identification and treatment of depression in ethnic elders are attitudes and behaviour of health professionals, their older ethnic patients, ethnic communities in general or some combination of the three.

Considerations in the assessment

To enable patients to feel comfortable and confident in explaining their symptoms, and thus facilitate exploration of potential mental health concerns, it is important to stress the confidential nature of the patient–doctor relationship and to ensure that patients are very clear that whatever is said during the consultation will not be discussed either within their 'community' or with their family members.

The following considerations should be given to consulting with an ethnic elder:

- When possible, use professional interpreters to facilitate doctor–patient communication ensuring that patients with depression are assessed in their native language.
- Where possible, avoid using family members as interpreters as this may discourage the patient from disclosing sensitive information, particularly as family tensions may be the root of the problem. The use of young children, as translators should also be avoided.
- Ideally translation is preferred to interpretation. In obtaining the information word for word as described by the patient loss of significant meanings is reduced. However subsequently it is advisable that the doctor should seek cultural interpretation of patients' problems as this may help in fully understanding the nature of presenting complaints.
- Consultation times may need to be extended when using translators to assist in communicating with the patient.
- Address the patient in the first person and not the interpreter during such consultations and remain attentive to the body language and facial expressions of the patient.

For detailed account of working with interpreters please see Phelan and Parkman (1995).

Learning to explore and explain depression in a culturally sensitive and appropriate way is the key to gaining patient trust and concordance. An understanding of language barriers and an appreciation of any hesitancy to discuss illness that is not of a physical nature are important in developing approaches that will assist in the identification of depressive disorder. The use of depression screening tools in native languages is useful in identifying the possibility of depression. However, for an appropriate treatment and management approach to be determined, further exploration and assessment of symptoms with the patient is required.

Depression screening scales for ethnic elders

Non-availability of reliable and valid measures of depression and the heterogeneity of the ethnic elderly population at times makes the use of screening scales difficult for the health professional.

The Geriatric Depression Scale (GDS) has been translated and validated for use in Hindi (Ganguli *et al.* 1999) and the English version has been validated for use in African-Caribbean elders (Rait *et al.* 1999). A validated Caribbean Culture-Specific Screen for emotional distress (CCSS) which performs similarly to the GDS is also available (Abas *et al.* 1998). Screening cut-off scores are discussed in Chapter 7.

Management issues

Pharmacological and psychological interventions

There is little research to support any particular pharmacological therapy being specifically beneficial for ethnic elders. The general considerations about prescribing antidepressants discussed in Chapter 2 should be followed but there is a particular need for detailed explanation about the basis for suggesting medication.

Similarly, there are no culturally sensitive psychological therapies available but again engaging the patient is critical. Abas and colleagues (1998), working in the African-Caribbean community, provide a helpful framework for these issues: (a) a courteous, respectful and warm manner, along with interest in ethnicity and country of origin; (b) flexibility about usual professional boundaries, for example, being prepared to share some experiences that facilitate rapport and acceptance of help; (c) not offering false promises; (d) offering a copy of written material; (e) comprehensive questions and not assuming that complaints or symptoms will be volunteered; (f) acknowledging losses, both recent and chronic, including racism. Rait in her commentary on Case 4.4 amplifies these areas.

Encouraging ethnic elders to attend community and faith-based groups organized by voluntary sector can often provide much-needed social support which they are used to but which is gradually eroding over time due to acculturation and changing family structure. Lambert addresses community resources in case commentary 7.

Working with the family

The social stigma of depression may cause families to deny or conceal the problem, or to delay or even fail to seek treatment. This warrants public education within a cultural framework, as well as collaborative efforts by the ethnic community and health-care providers. Particularly in ethnic elders from South Asia who still live in extended families it is important to keep the family 'on board'. This may seem difficult, as they may not share the viewpoint with the health provider on depression. So efforts to educate not only the patient, but also carers, become all the more important particularly regarding issues around medication use, side effects and time delay in symptom improvement.

REFERENCES

Abas M. A., Phillips C., Carter J., *et al.* (1998) Culturally sensitive validation of screening questionnaires for depression in older African-Caribbean people living in south London. *Br. J. Psychiatry* **173**, 249–54.

American Psychiatric Association (1994) *Diagnostic and Statistical Manual, Version IV.* Washington, DC: APA.

Beekman A. T. F., Deeg D. J. H., Van Tilburg T., *et al.* (1995) Major and minor depression in later life: a study of prevalence and risk factors. *J. Affect. Disord.* **36**, 65–75.

Bhatnagar K., Frank J. (1997) Psychiatric disorders in elderly from the Indian sub-continent living in Bradford. *Int. J. Geriatr. Psychiatry*; **12**, 907–12.

Bhopal R., Hayes L., White M., *et al.* (2002) Ethnic and socio-economic inequalities in coronary heart disease, diabetes and risk factors in Europeans and South Asians. *J. Publ. Health Med.* **24**, 95–105.

Blakemore K. (1982) Health and illness among the elderly of minority ethnic groups living in Birmingham: some new findings. *Health Trends* **14**, 69–72.

BMA and NHS Employers (2006) *Revisions to the GMS Contract, 2006/7: Delivering Investment in General Practice.* London: British Medical Association. 2006.

Burroughs H., Morley M., Lovell K., *et al.* (2006) 'Justifiable depression': how health professionals and patients view late-life depression – a qualitative study. *Fam. Practice* **23**, 369–377.

Chew-Graham C., Bashir C., Chantler K., Burman E., Batsleer J. (2002) South Asian women, psychological distress and self-harm: lessons for primary care trusts. *Health Soc. Care Commun.* **10**, 339–47.

Copeland J. R., Beekman A. T., Dewey A. T., *et al.* (1999) Depression in Europe: geographical distribution among older people. *Br. J. Psychiatry* **174**, 312–21.

Department of Health (1989) *Terms of Service for Doctors in General Practice.* London: HMSO.

Ganguli M., Dube S., Johnston J. M., *et al.* (1999) Depressive symptoms, cognitive impairment and functional impairment in a rural elderly population in India: a Hindi version of the geriatric depression scale (GDS-H). *Int. J. Geriatr. Psychiatry* **14**, 807–20.

Gerson S., Mistry R., Bastani R., *et al.* (2004) Symptoms of depression and anxiety (MHI) following acute medical/surgical hospitalisation and post discharge psychiatric diagnosis (DSM) in 839 geriatric US veterans. *Int. J. Geriatr. Psychiatry* **19**, 1155–67.

Good W. R., Vlachonikolis I., Griffiths R. A. (1987) The structure of depressive symptoms in the elderly. *Br. J. Psychiatry* **150**, 463–70.

Husain N., Creed F., Tomenson B. (1997) Adverse social circumstances and depression in people of Pakistani origin in the UK. *Br. J. Psychiatry* **171**, 434–8.

Hutchinson G., Gilvarry C. (1998) Ethnicity and dissatisfaction with mental health services. *Br. J. Psychiatry* **172**, 95–6.

Khan F., Waheed W. (2006) Suicide and selfharm in South Asian immigrants. In Gask L. (ed.) *Psychiatry*, vol. 5. London: Elsevier, pp. 283–5.

Kleinman A. (1987) Anthropology and psychiatry: the role of culture in cross-cultural research on illness. *Br. J. Psychiatry* **151**, 447–54.

Koffman J., Donaldson N., Hotopf M., Higginson I. J. (2005) Does ethnicity matter? Bereavement outcomes in two ethnic groups living in the United Kingdom. *Palliat. Support. Care* **3**, 183–90.

Krause I. B. (1989) Sinking heart: a Punjabi communication of distress. *Soc. Sci. Med.* **29**, 563–75.

Lawrence V., Banerjee S., Bhugra D., *et al.* (2006) Coping with depression in later life: a qualitative study of help-seeking in three ethnic groups. *Psychol. Med.* **36**, 1375–83.

Livingston G., Hawkins A., Graham N., *et al.* (1990) The Gospel Oak Study: prevalence rates of dementia, depression and activity limitation among elderly residents in Inner London. *Psychol. Med.* **20**, 137–46.

Marwaha S., Livingston G. (2002) Stigma, racism or choice: why do depressed ethnic elders avoid psychiatrists? *J. Affect. Disord.* **72**, 257–65.

McCracken C. F., Boneham M. A., Copeland J. R., *et al.* (1997) Prevalence of dementia and depression among elderly people in black and ethnic minorities. *Br. J. Psychiatry* **171**, 269–73.

Murray J., Williams P. (1986) Self-reported illness and general practice consultations in Asian-born and British-born residents of West London. *Soc. Psychiatry* **21**, 139–45.

Newman S. C., Sheldon C. T., Bland R. C. (1998) Prevalence of depression in an elderly community sample: a comparison of GMS-AGECAT and DSM IV diagnostic criteria. *Psychol. Med.* **28**, 1339–45.

NICE (2004) *Depression: Management of Depression in Primary and Secondary Care*, Clinical Guideline No. 23. London: National Institute for Health and Clinical Excellence.

Norman, A. (1985) *Triple Jeopardy: Growing Old in a Second Homeland*. London: Centre for Policy on Ageing.

Odell S. M., Surtees P. G., Wainwright N. W., Commander M. J., Sashidharan S. P. (1997) Determinants of general practitioner recognition of psychological problems in a multi-ethnic inner-city health district. *Br. J. Psychiatry* **171**, 537–41.

Osborn D. P., Fletcher A. E., Smeeth L., *et al.* (2003) Factors associated with depression in a representative sample of 14217 people aged 75 and older in the United Kingdom: results from the MRC trial of assessment and management of older people in the community. *Int. J. Geriatr. Psychiatry* **18**, 623–30.

Pearson S., Katzelnick D., Simon G., *et al.* (1999) Depression among high utilizers of medical care. *J. Gen. Intern. Med.* **14**, 461–8.

Phelan M., Parkman S. (1995) How to work with an interpreter. *Br. Med. J.* **311**, 555–7.

Prince M. J., Harwood R. H., Blizard R. A., *et al.* (1997) The Gospel Oak Project. V. Impairment, disability and handicap as risk factors for depression in old age. *Psychol. Med.* **2**, 311–21.

Rait G., Burns A., Chew C. A. (1996) Old age, ethnicity and mental illness: a triple whammy. *Br. Med. J.* **313**, 1347–8.

Rait G., Burns A., Baldwin R., *et al.* (1999) Screening for depression in older Afro-Caribbeans. *Fam. Practice* **16**, 591–5.

Regier D. A., Farmer M. E., Rae D. S., *et al.* (1993) One month prevalence of mental disorders in the United States and socio-demographic characteristics: the Epidemiological Catchment Area Study. *Acta Psychiatr. Scand.* **88**, 35–47.

Reynolds C. F., Perel J. M., Frank E., *et al.* (1999) Nortriptyline and interpersonal psychotherapy as maintenance therapies for recurrent major depression: a randomized controlled trial in patients older than 59 years. *J. Am. Med. Assoc.* **281**, 39–45.

Schaub R. T., Linden M., Copeland J. R. M. (2003) A comparison of GMS-A/AGECAT, DSM-III-R for dementia and depression, including sub threshold depression (SD): results from the Berlin Ageing Study (BASE). *Int. J. Geriatr. Psychiatry* **18**, 109–17.

Shah A., Dighe-Deo D. (1997) Elderly Gujeratis and psychogeriatics in a London psychogeriatric service. *Bull. Int. Psychogeriatr. Assoc.* **14**, 12–13.

Shah A., Lindesay J., Jagger C. (1998) Is the diagnosis of dementia stable over time among elderly immigrant Gujaratis in the United Kingdom. *Int. J. Geriatr. Psychiatry* **13**, 440–4.

Silveira E. R., Ebrahim S. (1998) Social determinants of psychiatric morbidity and well-being in immigrant elders and whites in east London. *Int. J. Geriatr. Psychiatry* **11**, 801–12.

United Kingdom National Census (2001) *National Statistics.* Available online at www.statistics.gov.uk/census2001/default/asp

Unützer J., Katon W., Sullivan M., Miranda J. (1999) Treating depressed older adults in primary care: narrowing the gap between efficacy and effectiveness. *Millbank Q.* **77**, 225–56.

Wilson K., Chen R., Taylor S., McCracken C. F. M., Copeland J. R. M. (1999a) Socio-economic deprivation, prevalence and prediction of depression in older community residents: the Liverpool MRC-Alpha study. *Br. J. Psychiatry* **175**, 549–53.

Wilson K., Copeland J. R. M., Donohue J., McCracken C. F. M. (1999b) The natural history of pharmacotherapy of older depressed community residents: the Liverpool ALPHA study. *Br. J. Psychiatry* **175**, 439–43.

World Health Organization (1980) *International Classification of Impairments Disabilities and Handicaps: A Manual of Classification Relating to the Consequences of Disease.* Geneva: WHO.

World Health Organization (1993) *The ICD-10 Classification of Mental and Behavioural Disorders: Research Criteria.* Geneva: WHO.

2

Management of late-life depression

Carolyn Chew-Graham, Robert Baldwin and Karina Lovell

Introduction

Most patients with depression are managed in primary care settings; however, a substantial number of patients are not recognized, and those who are diagnosed often do not receive effective treatment (Kessler *et al.* 1999). There is, however, a good evidence base for the management of depression in older people. Treatments that have been shown to work are the same as for younger adults: antidepressants, psychosocial and psychological interventions, or combinations of these and electroconvulsive treatment (ECT) for severe life-threatening or therapy-resistant cases. There is evidence to show that there are effective pharmacological (Wilson *et al.* 2001), psychological (Karel and Hinrichsen 2000) and psychosocial (Scogin and McElreath 1994) interventions for late-life depression, but these have yet to be adopted in primary care (Unützer 2002), in part because although cost-effective, they may involve added resource and investment to begin with. Only one in four depressed people receives effective pharmacological treatment and fewer than one in ten a talking therapy (Singleton *et al.* 2001). However, this is despite the fact that many people want and prefer 'talking treatments' (Rogers *et al.* 1993).

General principles of treatment

Goals of treatment

Table 2.1 provides a framework and summary of the goals for depression management (Baldwin *et al.* 2002).

Resolving all the symptoms of depression is the goal rather than getting the patient a bit better, as partial recovery is a predictor of future relapse. Current medication should be reviewed by the GP (primary care physician) at an early consultation, and any drugs that are not needed should be stopped after discussion with the patient. Polypharmacy increases the risk of depression

Integrated Management of Depression in the Elderly, ed. C. Chew-Graham, R. Baldwin and A. Burns. Published by Cambridge University Press. © Cambridge University Press 2008.

Table 2.1 Achieving management goals in depression in older people

Goal	Ways to achieve
Risk reduction – of suicide or harm from self-neglect	A risk assessment and monitoring of risk Prompt referral of urgent cases to a specialist
Remission of all depressive symptoms	Provision of appropriate treatment (usually an antidepressant and/or a psychological treatment) Giving the patient and his/her supporters timely education about depression and its treatment
To help the patient achieve optimal function	Enable practical support Ensure access to appropriate agencies which can help
To treat the whole person, including somatic problems	Treat co-existing physical health problems Reduce wherever possible the effects of handicap caused by factors such as chronic disease, sensory impairment and poor mobility Review medication and withdraw unnecessary ones
To prevent relapse and recurrence	Educate the patient about staying on medication once recovered Continuation treatment (staying on treatment after recovery; see text) Maintenance treatment (preventive treatment; see text)

and drug interactions, and increases the risk of poor concordance with taking tablets, including antidepressants. In addition, adherence to treatments is generally lower than average among depressed patients. It is particularly important to ask about over-the-counter medication and whether the patient has been self-medicating with St John's wort, if they have recognized depression as a problem themselves and tried to self-medicate.

The stepped care approach to the management of depression

Based on evidence of clinical effectiveness, cognitive behaviour therapy (CBT) is an appropriate psychological intervention for depression (Department of Health 2001). However, the demand for psychological therapies outstrips supply and psychological therapies in the UK are therefore characterized by relative inaccessibility and long patient waiting times (Lovell and Richards 2000). The adoption of a 'stepped care' system has been proposed to overcome these problems (Scogin *et al.* 2003). Stepped care for common mental health problems (Figure 2.1) is being introduced in the primary mental health care setting within the UK. The basic principle of stepped care is that patients presenting with a common mental health disorder will 'step through'

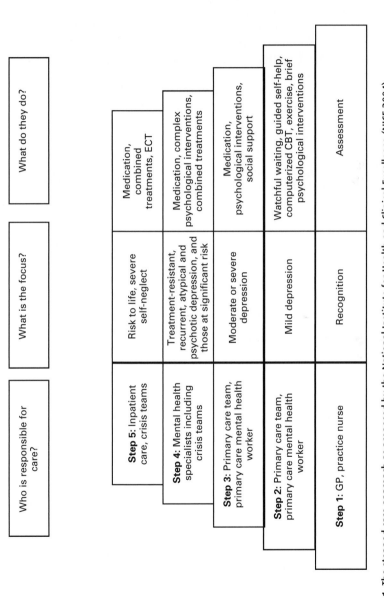

Who is responsible for care?	What is the focus?	What do they do?
Step 5: Inpatient care, crisis teams	Risk to life, severe self-neglect	Medication, combined treatments, ECT
Step 4: Mental health specialists including crisis teams	Treatment-resistant, recurrent, atypical and psychotic depression, and those at significant risk	Medication, complex psychological interventions, combined treatments
Step 3: Primary care team, primary care mental health worker	Moderate or severe depression	Medication, psychological interventions, social support
Step 2: Primary care team, primary care mental health worker	Mild depression	Watchful waiting, guided self-help, computerized CBT, exercise, brief psychological interventions
Step 1: GP, practice nurse	Recognition	Assessment

Figure 2.1 The stepped care approach as proposed by the National Institute for Health and Clinical Excellence (NICE 2004).

progressive levels of treatment as necessary, with the expectation that many of these patients will recover during the less intensive phases. Such a system seeks to enhance the efficiency and effectiveness of service delivery by providing low-intensity 'minimal interventions' to a proportion of patients in the first instance. The key features of stepped care are that treatment should be the least restrictive of effective therapies currently available and that the model is self-correcting. The definition of 'least restrictive' may refer to the impact on patients in terms of cost and personal inconvenience. In the context of publicly funded health-care systems, 'least restrictive' also often refers to the amount of specialist therapist time required (i.e. treatment intensity). More intensive treatments are reserved for patients who do not benefit from simpler first-line treatments, or for those who can be accurately predicted not to benefit from such treatments. The definition of 'self-correcting' means that the results of treatments and decisions about treatment provision are monitored system-atically, and changes are made ('stepping up') if current treatments are not achieving significant health gain. Thus, stepped care has the potential for deriving the greatest benefit from available therapeutic resources. The evidence base for stepped care, however, is limited (Bower and Gilbody 2005).

Self-help

The most appropriate 'minimal interventions' are those which are less depend-ent on the availability of therapists, and focus on patient-initiated use of evidence-based CBT techniques. One such minimal intervention is self-help. Self-help interventions are designed to provide effective care while reducing the need for input from specialist therapists, usually through 'health technol-ogies' such as bibliotherapy and computer programs. Treatments without therapist contact (so called 'pure self-help') are potentially the most efficient and could have the biggest impact on access, but these may not be optimally effective with depressed patients who lack motivation and confidence.

In the UK, the term 'guided self-help' is used to refer to self-help interven-tions with minimal therapist contact, which may provide the optimal balance between efficiency and effectiveness. The NICE Guidelines for depression propose the use of 'guided self-help' (GSH) at step 2, between 'watchful waiting' and brief psychological therapy, and defines GSH as involving a CBT-based self-help resource and limited support from a health-care profes-sional. The role of the health professional is to guide, support, review and monitor the patient's progress.

There is preliminary evidence that self-help interventions can be effective (McKendree-Smith *et al*. 2003, Anderson *et al*. 2005). However, evidence for the effectiveness of self-help interventions is not uniformly positive. Some studies have shown significant benefits (Proudfoot *et al*. 2004), whereas others have not (Richards *et al*. 2003, Mead *et al*. 2005). Despite the challenges posed, the use of GSH has been adopted successfully in primary care mental health services in the UK, and it has been shown that users and health professionals find the service acceptable and accessible (Lovell *et al.* 2006).

Implementing self-help

Lovell *et al.* (2006) describe the implementation of guided self-help for anxiety and depression in primary care:

- A patient-centred assessment focussing on the patient's main problem, including the autonomic, behavioural and cognitive aspects, impact of the problem on their work, social, private, family and life, risk assessment, expectations of treatment, social history, past mental health history and current use of drugs and alcohol.
- A formulation derived by discussion between the mental health worker and the patient ensuring that there was a 'shared understanding' of their current difficulties. Problem and goals (Marks 1986) derived by the patient and identification of the specific areas which the patient wished to work with.
- Standardized measures should be used to evaluate the process and outcome of the intervention are used including the Clinical Outcomes in Routine Evaluation–Outcome Measure (CORE–OM) (Barkham *et al.* 2001) and a range of specific disorder-related measures where appropriate.
- All patients are given a rationale for guided self-help, including an emphasis on self-management with the mental health worker as a facilitator rather than therapist.
- The patients are given written self-help materials (Kennedy and Lovell 2001) that are based on underlying CBT principles and include case histories using a range of interventions (relaxation, exposure therapy, cognitive restructuring, behavioural activation and problem-solving). Patients are encouraged to read the case histories and choose which intervention (or interventions) would benefit them most. Specific details of how to use the intervention are detailed within the manual along with relevant diaries.

Lovell describes the assessment as lasting 35–40 minutes with between three and six follow-up sessions (either face to face or by telephone) lasting 15–20 minutes. The facilitator's role is to review progress between sessions, support the patient to carry out the intervention, pre-empt difficulties that may arise, and engage in collaborative problem-solving as required.

Adapting such materials for the older person with depression has involved changing the case histories to make them more relevant to the older person, increasing the font size of the manual to enable ease of reading (Chew-Graham *et al.* 2007) and also recording the manual on tape for those with visual impairment or literacy difficulties.

Thus, despite some of potential problems of stepped care and guided self-help, it offers us a promising framework with which to reconfigure and deliver accessible, effective and acceptable psychological therapies. We need to ensure that older people experiencing common mental health problems such as depression and anxiety are not alienated or overlooked in the development of these models of care.

Practical considerations of the stepped care approach

In patients with mild/moderate depression, 'watchful waiting' is advocated with early review and consideration of the need for antidepressant or psychological therapy.

The stepped care approach stipulates that if there is expressed suicidality or risk of self-neglect, urgent referral to specialist old-age psychiatric services is required. If diagnosis is in doubt or there is a suspicion of psychotic features, referral to specialist old-age psychiatric services is also indicated.

If there is no risk of self-harm or self-neglect, at the initial consultation, the GP should provide education about depression for the patient and any carers present. Treatment of co-existing physical problems needs to be optimized. A discussion of social care needs (particularly loneliness and social isolation) is vital, with referral to social services or signposting to the voluntary sector as appropriate.

A plan of care should be agreed with the patient (and carers, if present) which should include agreement of goals of treatment, modalities of treatment and agreed review date. This plan should be reviewed and discussed with the patient at each consultation, and modified where necessary. It should be documented in the primary care records, with discussion with the patient of the usefulness of a patient-held plan.

The collaborative care approach

Most elderly people with depression in the UK will be managed in primary care and the lead clinician will be the GP or primary care physician. There is evidence, however, that other models of care which are protocol-driven and related to single-disease management may be more effective for the management of depression in older people. Thus, the collaborative care model has been developed to facilitate the management plan. The components include a depression care manager (usually a nurse, psychologist or social worker) who coordinates the care, including medication concordance. Built into the model is a requirement for regular dialogue between the primary care team and the specialist psychiatric services. The report of Unutzer et al. (2002) from the IMPACT study conducted in the USA is the largest to date. In this study 1801 depressed primary care patients (major depression, 17%; dysthymia, 30%; or both, 53%) were randomized to either usual care with active case management or usual care. At 12 months 45% of intervention patients achieved a 50%

reduction in symptoms compared to 19% of usual care subjects. There was a choice of problem-solving treatment (PST) or an antidepressant (prescribed by general practitioner). Another large study from the USA, using a similar model, found some effect in reducing suicidal thinking (Bruce *et al.* 2004). In the UK, this model has also recently been shown to be effective (Chew-Graham *et al.* 2007). In addition, the use of a collaborative care approach to the management of residents in nursing homes who are depressed has been shown to improve outcomes (Llewellyn-Jones *et al.* 1999, Procter *et al.* 1999.) In younger patients, compliance with medication improves when a collaborative care approach is utilized (Peveler and Kendrick 2001, von Korff and Goldberg 2001), and there is some evidence that concordance in older people is improved when such approaches are used (Llewellyn-Jones *et al.* 1999).

Pharmacotherapy

Initiating treatment with an antidepressant

The views of the patient (and carer) on tablets, and antidepressants in particular, need to be explored by the GP, and any myths (e.g. concerns about addictiveness) unearthed, discussed and dispelled. If the patient agrees to try an antidepressant, they can be involved in the choice of tablet. With so many antidepressants to choose from, it is important to match the antidepressant to the patient, taking account of tolerability, safety, side effects, drug interactions and contraindications, and previous patient experience of such drugs. For example, sertraline, citalopram and escitalopram are non-sedative and largely free from major interactions with other drugs. They are often preferred when frailty and risk of falling are concerns. Mirtazepine is sedative and may be helpful where insomnia is a prominent symptom. Tricyclic antidepressants (TCAs) have fallen out of favour largely on grounds of tolerability, safety and risk in overdose, but much of the early efficacy data comes from this class.

Involvement of the patient in decisions regarding treatment is a fundamental principle. The process of engagement in treatment is called 'concordance' to emphasize that good prescribing involves a relationship between patient and prescriber (Table 2.2). Patients may fail to take their antidepressants because of persistent attribution of all symptoms to physical illness. Time set aside to optimally manage current physical illness and to emphasize that depression too can be considered an illness, and that it is common, treatable and not a sign of moral weakness is time well spent. Reassurance is often needed that antidepressants are not addictive, and that depression is not 'senility' or a harbinger of dementia. Patients must be told not to expect immediate results and should be advised of commonly occurring side effects. Information sheets can help to back up discussion within the consultation. It is important to tell the

Table 2.2 Practical aspects of concordance in treatment

Understand patient's perception of what depression is
And that of his/her family and supporters
Explanation of what depression is
And what it is not (for example, 'weakness of character')
Clarify attribution of symptoms (for example, thinking that all symptoms are due to heart, bowels, etc.)
Explain side effects
Explain delay in onset
Agree management plan
Involve family/supporters if helpful and with patient's consent

patient not to stop the tablets once recovered. Usually antidepressants should be continued for up to 12 months after recovery, longer in recurrent depression.

The placebo response in clinical trials of depression is about 30%. This has caused interest in what may underlie 'non-specific' factors which promote recovery. Ones likely to be important are: having a plausible treatment delivered by someone perceived as having experience and knowledge, who is enthusiastic about it and takes depression seriously; the expectation of improvement; the positive regard of the prescriber towards the patient who is listened to with empathy and encourages him or her to verbalize their distress. These factors should never be underestimated.

Efficacy

Anderson *et al.* (2000) outline evidence-based guidelines for treating depressive disorders with antidepressants. A Cochrane Systematic Review of randomized controlled trials (RCTs) (Wilson *et al.* 2001) supports the efficacy of antidepressants over placebo in late-life major depression. The number-needed-to-treat (NNT: the number of subjects to be treated in order that one more will recover compared to no treatment) averaged between four and eight. This is as good as or indeed better as many medical treatments. In a further Cochrane Systematic Review of 29 studies there was no difference in efficacy between tricyclics and selective serotonin reuptake inhibitors (SSRIs) but tricyclics were associated with higher withdrawal rates due to side effects (Mottram *et al.* 2006).

There is weak evidence for the efficacy of antidepressants in depression complicating dementia (Bains *et al.* 2002). SSRIs are typically used but for milder depression 'watchful waiting' is appropriate as spontaneous recovery is common in the first few weeks after detection. Of particular importance in dementia is to consider care-givers who experience high rates of depression and whose depression 'rubs off' on the person with dementia.

The IMPACT study mentioned above (Callahan *et al.* 2005) and other research show that antidepressants are effective in patients who have a variety of physical disorders with their depression.

Table 2.3 provides an overview of main mode of action, principal side effects and doses for the main antidepressants.

Table 2.3 Side effect profiles and dosages of the main antidepressants used to treat late-life depression in the UK

Drug	Main mode of action	Main side effects	Starting dosage (mg)	Average daily dose (mg)
Amitriptyline	NA + + 5HT+	Sedation anticholinergic, postural hypotension, tachycardia/ arrhythmia	25–50	75–100
Imipramine	NA + + 5HT+	As for amitriptyline but less sedation	25	75–100
Nortripyline	NA + + 5HT+	As for amitriptyline but less sedation, anticholinergic effects and hypotension	10 tds	75–100
Dothiepin	NA + + 5HT+	As for amitriptyline	50–75	75
Mianserin	alpha-2 blocker	Sedation	30	30–90
Lofepramine	NA + + 5HT+	As for amitriptyline but less sedation, anticholinergic effects, hypotension and cardiac problems	70–140	70–210
Trazodone	$5HT_2$	Sedation, dizziness, headache	100	300
Citalopram	5HT	Nausea, vomiting, dyspepsia, abdominal pain, diarrhoea, headache, sexual dysfunction	20	20–40
Sertraline	5HT	As for citalopram	50	50–100
Fluoxetine	5HT	As for citalopram but insomnia and agitation more common	20	20
Paroxetine	5HT	As for citalopram but sedation and anticholinergic effects may occur	20	20
Fluvoxamine	5HT	As for citalopram but nausea more common	50–100	100–200

Table 2.3 (*cont.*)

Drug	Main mode of action	Main side effects	Starting dosage (mg)	Average daily dose (mg)
Escitalopram	5HT	As for citalopram	5	10–20
Moclobemide	MAO	Sleep disturbance, nausea, agitation	300	300–400
Venlafaxine	NA 5HT	Nausea, insomnia, dizziness, dry mouth, somnolence, hyper- and hypotension	75	150
Duloxetine	NA 5HT	Nausea, insomnia, dizziness	30	60
Mirtazepine	alpha-2 blocking selective antagonist, $5HT_2$ and $5HT_3$ receptors	Increased appetite, weight gain, somnolence, headache	15	30

5HT, serotonin; MAO, monoamine oxidase; NA, noradrenaline; tds, three times a day.

Side effects of medication

Side effects are the commonest reason for poor adherence to antidepressant medication (Mitchell 2006).

Anticholinergic side effects include dry mouth, blurred vision, constipation, urinary retention and cardiotoxicity (so that an electrocardiogram (ECG) may be needed prior to starting an older TCA). Persistent dryness of the mouth, another anticholinergic effect, can lead to dental caries. These effects are common with TCAs and cardiac arrhythmia in overdose can be fatal. Delirium is a possibility and is more likely in patients who are have co-morbid physical illnesses. Postural hypotension due to adrenergic blockade is a serious problem with TCAs and histaminic effects often cause sedation and, in the longer term, weight gain. Lofepramine is a second-generation TCA which is less likely to cause these adverse effects.

The SSRIs lack cardiotoxicity and are not lethal in overdose, but they have undesirable side effects. These include nausea (around 15%), diarrhoea (around 10%), insomnia (5–15%), anxiety and/or agitation (2–15%), sexual dysfunction (up to 30% among younger people treated, unknown prevalence in elderly patients), headache and, occasionally, weight loss. The main metabolite of fluoxetine is clinically active and remains so for approximately a week, possibly longer for older patients. The SSRIs have minimal impact on cognitive function in older patients with depression and there is also evidence that SSRIs and lofepramine cause less impairment than the older tricyclics in cognitive skills relevant to driving. There is growing concern about gastrointestinal haemor-rhage in patient prescribed SSRIs, particularly elderly patients (van Walraven *et al.* 2001). Caution should be exercised in patients treated with non-steroidal anti-inflammatory drugs (NSAIDs) or aspirin. Epilepsy is a caution for the use of antidepressants as these drugs may reduce the seizure threshold.

Discontinuation symptoms may occur with all classes of antidepressants if they are abruptly stopped after several weeks of treatment. They are more common and severe with antidepressants that have a short half-life. Paroxetine seems to cause this more than other SSRIs.

Moclobemide is well tolerated by older people. Although a special diet is not required, patients should be aware of the drug interactions with painkillers and other antidepressants. Co-prescriptions of tricyclic and SSRIs should be avoided in primary care. Venlafaxine is generally well tolerated among older patients, particularly if the dose is increased slowly. The main side effects are nausea and gastrointestinal disturbance but blood pressure regulation can be problematic (so blood pressure should be monitored regularly). Duloxetine, a newer dual-acting antidepressant, does not appear to be cardiotoxic although initial nausea can be a problem. Mirtazepine has some side effects similar to tricyclics. Weight gain and sedation can be troublesome, although the latter can be beneficial where insomnia is prominent.

Although commonly asserted, it is probably not true that older patients take longer to recover than younger ones, provided that correct dosages are used. If there is little or no improvement (equal to or less than 25% on a recognized mood rating scale, for example) by week 4 then recovery or remission is unlikely. If, however, recovery has started, then optimizing the dosage and continuing the drug results in more patients recovering. Mottram *et al.* (2002) showed that of those eventually recovered, 61% had done so by six weeks and 88% by eight weeks.

Patients who do not respond

If, at four weeks, there has been little or no response to an antidepressant given in adequate dosage and where concordance has been achieved, then recovery is unlikely. In this case, if the dose given is sub-therapeutic (e.g. TCAs and some SSRIs) then the dose can be increased. If the dose has been therapeutic, then it is sensible to discuss with the patient changing the antidepressant to a drug from a different class (see Box 2.1).

Patients with resistant depression (typically patients who do not respond to two consecutive antidepressant drugs in optimum dose for at least four weeks each) should be referred to a specialist old-age psychiatrist (according to the stepped care approach), as should patients with high suicide risk or possible

---

Box 2.1 The poorly responsive patient

- If little or no response by four weeks
  - increase the dose or change to another antidepressant class
- If limited response
  - increase dose (if not already optimal), or continue for a further two to four weeks, refer to specialist for consideration for augmentation (which may be with medication or a psychological intervention)
- Ensure psychological treatments offered
- If no response after further four weeks
  - refer to old-age psychiatrist

Box 2.2 Indications for ECT

- Patient actively suicidal
- Urgent treatment to prevent deterioration in health in cases of self-neglect
- Psychotic depression
- Inadequate response to two trials of medication and/or failure of augmentation of treatment
- Intolerance of medication
- Prior good response

---

underlying dementia or when the diagnosis is in doubt. At this stage, the specialist will consider the use of augmentation regimens (using two antidepressants and/or a mood stabilizer) or ECT (Box 2.2) (NICE 2004). Augmentation can be with medication or a psychological intervention. As is emphasized by our international commentaries in later chapters, it is frequently the case that psychological interventions are only available following a referral to local specialist psychiatric services.

Sources of treatment variability in older patients

Altered pharmacokinetics, different pharmacodynamics, a greater chance of polypharmacy and hence drug interactions and reduced compensatory mechanisms are all important factors which bear upon treatment response to antidepressants in older adults. An overview of these is provided in Lotrich and Pollock (2005) and the most important 'bottom line' is that inter-individual difference in drug handling is greater than in younger adults – the same dose may have less predictable effects. There is a greater chance of side effects in older people. Examples include anticholinergic effects with TCAs and paroxetine, treatment-emergent parkinsonism with SSRIs and possibly a higher chance of developing the syndrome of inappropriate antidiuretic hormone secretion (SIADH) which can dangerously lower the sodium in the blood causing unpleasant symptoms, some of which are similar to depressive disorder. Reduced homoeostatic reserve can lead to impaired orthostatic responses, impaired thermoregulation, a greater risk of delirium and an increased risk of falls, the latter *not* being confined to the older TCAs.

Psychological interventions

Cognitive behavioural therapy (CBT), inter-personal psychotherapy (IPT), problem-solving treatment (PST) and psychodynamic psychotherapy are the most widely researched forms of psychotherapy in later-life depression (Gatz *et al.* 1998, Pinquart and Sorensen 2001). CBT addresses the faulty logic that often accompanies depression, IPT emphasizes relational issues, for example loss, inter-personal functioning and role transitions, while PST deals with the here and now, focussing on current difficulties and setting future goals. Psychodynamic techniques use the relationship with the therapist to explore transference dynamics from earlier developmental stages which impinge on the present. Some of the techniques have been used in elderly people in a group setting to good effect, with the additional advantage of overcoming social isolation as seen in the second UK case commentary (see Case 3.2).

In moderate to severe (non-psychotic) depressive episodes, combining antidepressant medication with a psychological intervention such as CBT or IPT is associated with better outcomes than either intervention alone (Reynolds *et al.* 1999).

Anxiety management can be a highly effective adjunctive treatment for depressed patients, especially where patients who are recovering from depression are left with residual anxiety, low confidence or phobic avoidance which can undermine functional improvement. Techniques may include progressive relaxation, either alone with a commercial tape, or in groups. The setting of graded tasks under the supervision of an occupational therapist, nurse or psychologist can be extremely helpful.

Exercise and activity are important both to avoid depression and counter it. Behavioural activation is a technique which can overcome the withdrawal and apathy that so often exists in late-life depression. It works by helping the patient develop a schedule of activities, agreed with the patient with or without a written diary to support implementation (see Chapter 7 for more detail).

The GP can use some of these techniques within the primary care consultation, particularly advising about diet, exercise and alcohol, encouraging behaviour change and goal-setting, challenging negative thinking and teaching relaxation techniques. Most GPs have access to self-help leaflets which can be given to patients to reinforce the content of discussion within consultations.

Important too is family work. The patient may unconsciously use the family to foster invalidism which the family may then unwittingly reinforce. The unconscious goal may be to live under the same roof as one's children. More positively the family is often critical in ensuring a successful outcome in treatment, for example reinforcing messages about treatment concordance, exercise and activity, goal-setting, etc.

Social interventions

Poor housing, poverty, high local rates of crime or fear of crime and other indices of deprivation are important determinants of depression. Many factors interact: low socio-economic status is linked to poverty, poor housing, higher exposure to crime and poorer health. Sometimes a change to better circumstances can be crucial to recovery. Generally though it is best to defer discussion of issues such as rehousing until after recovery of depression as the patient's view may alter. The impact of these factors will also be affected by other ones such as social support and individual coping styles. Interventions for each of these can be addressed as part of recovering from depression.

Handicap, the social disadvantage arising out of a disability, is intimately linked to depression in older adults. Social workers can help address some sources of handicap and 'signpost' the patient with depression to resources which may help reduce this and other disadvantages. Day centres, luncheon clubs and resource centres, some designed for particular minority groups, can be helpful in countering the isolation which may be either a cause or consequence of depression.

REFERENCES

Anderson I. M., Nutt D. J., Deakin J. F. (2000) Evidence-based guidelines for treating depressive disorders with antidepressants: revision of the 1993 British Association for Psychopharmacology Guidelines. *J. Psychopharmacology* **14**, 3–20.

Anderson L., Lewis G., Araya R., *et al.* (2005). Self-help books for depression: how can practitioners and patients make the right choice? *Br. J. Gen. Practice* **55**, 387–92.

Bains J., Birks J. S., Dening T. D. (2002) Antidepressants for treating depression in dementia. *Cochrane Database of Systematic Reviews*, Issue 4.

Baldwin R. C., Chiu E., Katona C., Graham N. (2002) *Guidelines on Depression in Older People: Practising the Evidence.* London: Martin Dunitz.

Barkham M., Margison F., Leach C., *et al.* (2001) Service profiling and outcomes benchmarking using the CORE-OM: towards practice-based evidence in the psychological therapies. *J. Consult. Clin. Psychol.*, **69**, 184–96.

Bower P., Gilbody S. (2005) Stepped care in psychological therapies: access, effectiveness and efficiency – narrative literature review. *Br. J. Psychiatry* **186**, 11–17.

Bruce M. L., Have T. R. T., Reynolds C. F., *et al.* (2004) Reducing suicidal ideation and depressive symptoms in depressed older primary care patients: a randomized controlled trial. *J. Am. Med. Assoc.*, **291**, 1081–91.

Callahan C. M., Kroenke K., Counsell S. R., *et al.* for the IMPACT Investigators (2005) Treatment of depression improves physical functioning in older adults. *J. Am. Geriatr. Soc.* **53**, 367–73.

Chew-Graham C. A., Lovell K., Roberts C., *et al.* (2007) A randomized controlled trial to test the feasibility of a collaborative care model for the management of depression in older people. *Br. J. Gen. Practice* **57** 364–70.

Department of Health (2001) *Treatment Choice in Psychological Therapies and Counselling: Evidence-based Clinical Practice Guideline.* London: HMSO.

Gatz M., Fiske A., Fox L. S., *et al.* (1998) Empirically validated psychological treatments for older adults. *J. Ment. Health Aging* **4**, 9–46.

Karel M. J., Hinrichsen G. (2000) Treatment of depression in late life: psychotherapeutic interventions. *Clin. Psychol. Rev.* **20**, 707–29.

Kennedy A., Lovell K. (2001) *What Should I do? Depression and Anxiety.* Southampton, UK: RTFB Publishing.

Kessler D., Lloyd K., Lewis G., *et al.* (1999) Cross-sectional study of symptom attribution and recognition of depression and anxiety in primary care. *Br. Med. J.* **318**, 436–40.

Llewellyn-Jones R. H., Balkie K. A., Smithers H., *et al.* (1999) Multifaceted shared care intervention for late-life depression in residential care: randomized controlled trial. *Br. Med. J.* **319**, 676–82.

Lotrich F. E., Pollock B. G. (2005) Aging and clinical pharmacology: implications for antidepressants. *J. Clin. Pharmacol.* **45**, 1106–22.

Lovell K., Richards D. (2000) Multiple Access Points and Levels of Entry (MAPLE): ensuring choice, accessibility and equity for CBT services. *Behav. Cognit. Psychother.* **28**, 379–91.

Lovell K., Bee P., Richards D., Kendal S. (2006) Evaluating service provision in an urban primary care setting. *Prim. Health Care Res. Devel.* **7**, 211–20.

Marks I. M. (1986) *Behavioural Psychotherapy: Maudsley Pocketbook of Clinical Management.* Bristol, UK: Wright.

McKendree-Smith N., Floyd M., Scogin F. (2003) Self-administered treatments for depression: a review. *J. Clin. Psychol.* **59**, 275–88.

Mead N., MacDonald W., Bower P., *et al.* (2005) The clinical effectiveness of guided self-help versus waiting list control in the management of anxiety and depression: a randomized controlled trial. *Psychol. Med.* **35**, 1633–43.

Mitchell A. J. (2006) Two-week delay in onset of action of antidepressants: new evidence. *Br. J. Psychiatry* **188**, 105–6.

Mottram P. G., Wilson K. C., Ashworth L., Abou-Saleh M. (2002) The clinical profile of older patients' response to antidepressants: an open trial of sertraline. *Int. J. Geriatr. Psychiatry* **17**, 574–8.

Mottram P., Wilson K., Strobl J. (2006) Antidepressants for depressed elderly. *Cochrane Database of Systematic Reviews*, Issue 1.

NICE (2004) *Depression: Management of Depression in Primary and Secondary Care*, Clinical Guideline No. 23. London: National Institute for Health and Clinical Excellence.

Peveler R., Kendrick T. (2001) Treatment delivery and guidelines in primary care. *Br. Med. Bull.* **57**, 193–206.

Pinquart M., Sorensen S. (2001) How effective are psychotherapeutic and other psychosocial interventions with older adults? A meta-analysis. *J. Ment. Health Aging* **7**, 207–43.

Procter R., Burns A., Stratton Powell H., *et al.* (1999) Behavioral management in nursing and residential homes: a randomized controlled trial. *Lancet* **354**, 26–9.

Proudfoot J., Ryden C., Everitt B., *et al.* (2004) Clinical efficacy of computerized cognitive-behavioural therapy for anxiety and depression in primary care: randomized controlled trial. *Br. J. Psychiatry* **185**, 46–54.

Reynolds C. F. III, Frank F., Perel J. M., *et al.* (1999) Nortriptyline and interpersonal psychotherapy as maintenance therapies for recurrent major depression: a randomized controlled trial in patients older than 59 years. *J. Am. Med. Assoc.* **281**, 39–45.

Richards A., Barkham M., Cahill J., *et al.* (2003) PHASE: a randomized, controlled trial of supervised self-help cognitive behavioural therapy in primary care. *Br. J. Gen. Practice* **53**, 764–70.

Rogers A., Pilgrim D., Lacey R. (1993) *Experiencing Psychiatry: Users' Views of Services.* Basingstoke, UK: Macmillan.

Scogin F., McElreath L. (1994) Efficacy of psychosocial treatments for geriatric depression: a quantitative review. *J. Consult. Clin. Psychol.* **62**, 69–74.

Scogin F., Hanson A., Welsh D. (2003) Self-administered treatment in stepped-care models of depression treatment. *J. Clin. Psychol.* **59**, 341–9.

Singleton N., Bumpstead R., O'Brien M., Lee A., Meltzer H. Y. (2001) *Office of National Statistics: Psychiatric Morbidity among Adults Living in Private Households, 2000.* London: HMSO.

Unützer J (2002) Diagnosis and treatment of older adults with depression in primary care. *Biol. Psychiatry* **52**, 285–92.

Unützer J., Katon W., Callahan C. M., *et al.* (2002) Collaborative care management of late life depression in the primary care setting. *J. Am. Med. Assoc.* **288**, 2836–45.

von Korff M., Goldberg D. (2001) Improving outcomes in depression. *Br. Med. J.* **323**, 948–9.

van Walraven C., Mamdani M., Wells, P. (2001) Inhibition of serotonin reuptake by antidepressants and upper gastrointestinal bleeding in elderly patients: retrospective cohort study. *Br. Med. J.* **323**, 655–8.

Wilson K., Mottram P., Sivanranthan A., Nightingale A. (2001) Antidepressant versus placebo for depressed elderly. *Cochrane Database of Systematic Reviews*, Issue 2.

3

Management of late-life depression in primary care: case studies UK

In order to illustrate the integrated management of depression in older people in UK primary care, we asked contributors to provide commentaries on a selection of cases drawn from real-life scenarios. The following three chapters contain these commentaries together with a summary by the editors. The first three cases illustrate the management of patients with mild to moderate depressive symptoms in primary care.

Case 3.1 A request for sleeping tablets

Mr Seth Y, aged 69 years, presents to his GP complaining that he can't sleep. He admits to feeling upset and worried, although he doesn't know why. He denies that anything has recently happened to him, but the practice receptionist is aware that his son and family have emigrated to New Zealand, and both Mr and Mrs Y have admitted to the staff at the desk that they miss their grandchildren. He comes to see the GP to ask for some sleeping tablets.

Mr SY doesn't often attend the practice, he has been on Losartan for hypertension for five years and his recent review with the nurse (including cholesterol and renal function) was satisfactory.

Please describe the assessment of Mr SY in the GP consultation. Discuss the options available for the management of the patient. Besides medication, what strategies are available for the management of Mr SY's insomnia?

Dr Ceri Dornan, General Practitioner and GP with Special Interest (Mental Health), Manchester Primary Care Trust
Mr SY does not attend surgery frequently, so his request for sleeping tablets would seem unusual and arouse my curiosity. As I observe him coming in, I have the opportunity to note his body language, facial expression, degree of self-care and physical comfort when walking and sitting down. He may be hesitant about making his request and an open style of consultation would be

Integrated Management of Depression in the Elderly, ed. C. Chew-Graham, R. Baldwin and A. Burns.
Published by Cambridge University Press. © Cambridge University Press 2008.

helpful to allow him to find words to express himself. He has spoken of his feelings of missing his family with reception staff, a valuable source of background intelligence in general practice, where patients may share personal details they would not see as relevant to discuss with their GP. I would wonder whether his insomnia was related to his worries, whether he was becoming depressed and if he had any physical causes of insomnia making his threshold for waking lower. His wife's pattern of sleeping would be relevant, as she is likely to be responding to the family situation as well.

Some people are irritated by an exploration by the GP of their request for sleeping tablets rather than just receiving a prescription, so it can help to share the above thoughts and indicate a willingness to find a solution to the sleeping problem. The order in which the areas are explored will depend on the person. This man may not be used to talking about his feelings, so discussing physical symptoms first could help to develop rapport.

Common physical causes of insomnia in a man of his age would be urinary frequency from prostate enlargement, pain from osteoarthritis and breathlessness from heart or lung problems. I would note his normal renal function from his recent hypertension check and review the medication he was taking, to check if in addition to Losartan, he was having diuretics or a beta-blocker for his hypertension, as they can cause sleep problems. General questions about weight and appetite contribute to assessment of his physical and mental wellbeing and can lead onto enquiry about his mood. The screening questions for depression recommended in the NICE Guidelines (NICE 2004a), now introduced into the annual review for people with diabetes and heart disease as part of the GP Contract (BMA and NHS Employers 2006), are a suitable start. They can be introduced by a comment that sometimes sleep problems are related to our mood:

'Over the last month, have you often been bothered by feeling down, depressed or hopeless?'
and
'Over the last month, have you often been bothered by having little interest or pleasure in doing things?'

A positive response to either or both questions lead to a further assessment of symptoms to confirm if he is depressed and if so, how severe this is using one of the tools recommended for primary care (such as the PHQ-9). Sometimes going through the questions on an assessment tool can help the person to connect the symptoms they are experiencing to the possibility that they are in fact depressed. In a older patient it may be better to go through any schedule used, rather than ask him to complete it on his own. The tools include a question about suicidal thoughts, but I would check this out further through discussion, possibly by asking what he thought about when he couldn't sleep and whether he ever felt hopeless about the future or that life was not worth living. It would be important to remind myself of any past psychiatric history and previous response to losses in his life, and to ask about his alcohol and tobacco consumption. He has recently had a review of his blood pressure with the practice nurse, but I would consider further physical examination depending on symptoms obtained from the history, perhaps a prostate assessment, chest and heart examination and any painful joints. Investigations would follow from any positive findings. Sometimes a lead into more personal questions can be initiated during a physical examination, e.g. 'How is your son getting on?' as he is getting dressed. This can open an exploration of his feelings about the emigration, fears about the ability of himself and his wife to travel a long distance, maybe feelings of being abandoned. I would want to know about his day-to-day activities, interests, involvement in any religious faith and other supports from family and friends. His presenting concern was insomnia, which is probably part of an adjustment reaction to his son's move. By making this link for him, the process of adjustment to loss can be discussed, using the example of bereavement. I would encourage him to share feelings with his wife, who is likely to be feeling the same, and explore his usual coping strategies when faced with worries. Behavioural and self-help strategies to deal with insomnia, backed up with written information, can be given by the GP or primary care nurse (as discussed by Helen Pusey: see next section). If his symptoms have been present for more than a few weeks, he could be offered information about local counselling services, for example, some branches of Age Concern offer services. There may be a mental health worker available to the surgery to offer guided self-help or brief therapy to deal with depressive symptoms and support activity to reduce their impact. A follow-up appointment to continue monitoring for depression should be offered (and this is in accordance with NICE guidance (NICE 2004a) which recommends 'watchful waiting' in the initial management of mild to moderate depression), and there will be an opportunity for the practice nurse to monitor his mood when he next attends for blood pressure review. Ideally the practice will have a policy in place which sets out the actions a practice nurse should take if she identifies someone as depressed.

Would medication be appropriate? He is not likely to be sufficiently depressed to merit antidepressants, unless he had a serious depression in the past, particularly in response to loss, when early introduction of an antidepressant might be advisable. I would, however, take into account his score on any schedule used. An explanation of the risks of taking sleeping tablets, with risk of dependency, falls, loss of concentration and effects on driving ability, may be enough to satisfy him that this is not the appropriate action. If he is insistent, clearly very tired, or using alcohol to sleep, a decision must be made whether refusal to prescribe will lose an opportunity to engage him in follow-up. A compromise may be to offer a brief, seven to ten days, course of a mild hypnotic, e.g. Temazepam 10 mg, with advice about driving and alcohol and indication that this will not be repeated. Active follow-up should be offered. There should be an agreement in the practice over use of hypnotics, so if he returned to see a different partner, he would receive a consistent message. A clear plan of management in the notes is helpful in this situation. There is a risk that this man will not adjust to his son's move, coming at a time when he will have had expectations of how his life might be. His wife may be feeling the same. Positive engagement and follow-up by practice team members at any contact with the couple are an important part of reducing this risk.

Helen Pusey, Lecturer in Nursing, University of Manchester
There have been calls for primary care nurses to play a greater role in the detection and management of depression for at least 10 years (Katona *et al.* 1995, Banerjee *et al.* 1996), and in England, the National Service Framework for Older People (NSFOP) (Department of Health 2001) reiterates this expectation. The NSFOP clearly identifies that older people with depression are likely to be assessed and treated entirely within primary care. This suggests all members of the primary care team will have a role within this process and thus nurses should be equipped with core skills in mental health enabling them to assess, provide appropriate advice and manage mild depression.

District nurses are in a prime position to play a major part in detection and management of depression in older people as 62% of their caseload is aged 65 or over (Audit Commission 1999). In addition, half the community-based population aged over 85 are on a district nurse caseload (Audit Commission 1999).

Assessment

Patient-centred assessment is the first step that allows the nurse to understand the problem and the effect it is having on the person's life. It can incorporate a number of components including a measurable screening tool and a risk assessment. For a successful assessment the nurse must also engage the patient utilizing effective communication skills; for example, demonstrate interest, establish the patient's expectations, show empathy and listen appropriately.

If this was the initial contact the district nurse would undertake a full biopsychosocial assessment as part of their First Assessment. However, if Mr SY was already on the district nurse caseload, a modified assessment would take place, incorporating the knowledge already gathered. This presenting problem would be assessed across the following domains:

- Eliciting Mr SY's perspective
- Assessing mood and eliciting symptoms of depression
- Assessing physical problems that might be affecting mood
- Assessing social networks and social supports
- Assessing risk.

Eliciting Mr SY's perspective

With a patient-centred assessment it is important to identify how Mr SY feels about his situation. What does Mr SY think the problem is and what does he think would help?

Assessing mood and eliciting symptoms of depression

The ABC model of emotion can be utilized to help the patient and the nurse reach common understanding of the patient's feelings. The model breaks down the feeling or emotion into its components parts. 'A' represents the autonomic and other physical symptoms, 'B' represents behaviour and 'C' represents cognitions or thoughts. These elements are linked and the nurse can demonstrate how they impact on each other. For example Mr SY's sadness could be considered as:

A: Difficulty sleeping.

B: Not participating in as many social activities.

C: Thinking 'My grandchildren will forget who I am.'

As part of the assessment it would be helpful to utilize a screening tool. Although short item tools such as the 4-item Geriatric Depression Scale (D'Ath 1994) will provide a valid and reliable indicator of possible depression, use of a longer tool such as the 15-item Geriatric Depression Scale (Shiekh and Yesavage 1986) would provide a useful baseline to monitor progress and provide tangible feedback to Mr SY.

Assessing physical problems

Certain physical illness, nutritional deficiencies or medications can trigger or exacerbate low mood. If appropriate the district nurse would refer Mr SY to the GP to eliminate any physical factors that might be affecting his mood.

Assessing risk

Mr SY's risk of suicide should be considered. Although we do not have any information on his long-term risk factors we do know that he has short-term ones: he is an older male and there are precipitating factors such as that he has recent separation from his family. In addition it is known that older people who commit suicide are likely to have contacted primary care within a month before their death. Once rapport has been established the district nurse should ask appropriate questions to assess the level of risk.

Management

As Mr SY's problem appears to be a mild lowering of mood in response to a change in his social circumstances, it would be appropriate for the district nurse to provide management. Currently, Mr SY would be considered on step 2 of the stepped care approach (see Chapter 2). At this stage the most appropriate management will be 'watchful waiting' and general advice with a follow up assessment in two weeks.

The general advice would cover the following:

- Sleep hygiene. Here the district nurse can provide Mr SY with appropriate education about strategies to promote good sleep habits such as getting sufficient bright light during the day, keeping a regular sleep schedule, not spending too much time in bed, avoiding drinks, especially caffeine, in the hours before bedtime and ensuring the bedroom is the correct temperature.
- Increasing pleasant activities. When people experience low mood they may stop or reduce the amount of activity they undertake and this reduction in activity can make them feel more depressed. Mr SY could be encouraged to plan enjoyable and realistic activities thus helping to improve his mood.
- Strategies for maintaining contact with family. The loss of regular contact with his grandchildren is an obvious concern for Mr SY. The district nurse could suggest ways that he might enhance his contact, for example by having a regular time for a phone call or installing a webcam to enable them to see each other.

Appropriate referral

If there was no improvement in Mr SY's mood or if his symptoms appear to deteriorate, or if he expressed thoughts of self-harm, it would be appropriate for the district nurse to refer him to the GP, with an indication of the degree of urgency when making this referral. Depending on local protocols it might also be appropriate to send a referral to the primary care mental health team or secondary care community mental health team if the district nurse feels Mr SY is at risk or if his symptoms become serious or complex. The community mental health team should also be available to provide the district nurse with advice should there be any concerns regarding the assessment and management of Mr SY.

The district nurse will also have the option of signposting Mr SY to other suitable agencies or services, particularly voluntary agencies, depending on his needs. For example if Mr SY had limited social contact outside the family, the district nurse could suggest local groups or organizations that would provide opportunities to enhance his networks.

There are, however, barriers to the involvement of the district nurse in the identification and appropriate management of patients with depression. In common with other non-mental-health specialists in primary care there is a risk of therapeutic nihilism, the belief that there is very little that can be offered to this group coupled with the perception that depression is an understandable consequence of ageing, isolation or poor social conditions (Burroughs et al. 2006). This can be compounded by the tendency of older people to present with somatic symptoms, and a reluctance to disclose low mood or take up the nurse's time.

The main focus of the district nurse is managing physical health, with depression not necessarily regarded as part of the remit. The majority of district nurses will have a general nursing background with very limited, if any, mental health training. This potentially leaves them feeling ill-equipped to address depression. There can be a perception that asking questions to do with mood will open a 'Pandora's box' they may not have the skills or time to deal with. In addition, apart from referring to the GP for antidepressants the district nurse may feel there is little to offer. Despite evidence of effectiveness there has been lack of psychological therapies available to older people with many services only open to those under 65. Unfortunately the latest Department of Health initiative *Improving Access to Psychological Therapies* (Department of Health 2006) is unlikely to improve this situation as the focus is on facilitating return to work and excludes older people.

Although overcoming these barriers will require a co-ordinated approach across primary care, there is potential for district nurses to receive appropriate training enabling them to assess mood within a reasonable time frame and offer general support and advice.

Case 3.2 Loneliness and grief

Mrs Winifred E is a 72-year-old lady who had been married for 49 years when her husband died last Christmas from lung cancer after a very short period of illness. She now lives alone, although sees her daughter every week and her son (who lives 200 miles away) occasionally. Her neighbours often take her shopping but the whole street has been upset by a spate of recent burglaries. Mrs WE has had her shed broken into and her kitchen window broken, so she feels very frightened in her home, especially at night. She misses her husband dreadfully and blames herself for not noticing the signs of ill-health. She feels he would have known how to deal with the threat of being burgled, and she is angry with him for leaving her alone.

Mrs WE has hypothyroidism and takes thyroxine 100 µg daily. Her last thyroid function tests were normal. She had a peptic ulcer in the past (confirmed by gastroscopy in 1984) and takes lansoprazole. Her GP records reveal that she had an episode of postnatal depression after her youngest child (her son) was born and which was treated with amitriptyline. She does not appear to have been treated for depression since that time.

She attends the practice nurse for her flu vaccine and admits that she is upset and worried and having difficulty sleeping. The nurse suggests that she could attend a local lunch club and also gives her some information on protecting her house. She suggests that she should see the GP, but Mrs WE replies that she doesn't want to bother her and anyway doesn't 'like the thought of tablets'. Mrs WE does, however, attend the appointment that the nurse encouraged her to make, but starts by saying 'I don't know why I'm here, you can't do anything.'

Please describe the assessment of Mrs WE in the GP consultation. Discuss the options available for the management of the patient. If medication is thought to be appropriate, discuss choice of drug and also how Mrs WE's reluctance to take medication could be addressed.

Professor Christopher Dowrick, General Practitioner and Professor of Primary Care, University of Liverpool

Assessment

Mrs WE has several interrelated problems. The most important one is the recent death of her husband. She lives in an unsafe local environment, and may be socially isolated, and she has at least one long-term medical condition.

Grief, complicated grief or depression?

With regard to the impact of her husband's death 10 months ago, my main concern is to decide whether Mrs WE is going through a normal grief reaction, or whether she fulfils criteria for either a complicated grief reaction or a depressive disorder. Although the diagnostic boundaries between these apparently discrete conditions are far from clear (Dowrick 2004), it is important to consider them since they predict different treatment options.

Grief is intense and painful but, unfortunately, an inevitable part of the human experience (Murray Parkes 1998). It often includes: a sense of disbelief, shock, numbness and feelings of unreality, particularly in the first few weeks; longing for and preoccupation with the loved one, and thoughts of wanting to die or join them (but not suicidal plans or attempts); feelings of anger or guilt; sadness and tearfulness; disturbed sleep and appetite and occasionally weight loss; and seeing or hearing the voice of the deceased. These experiences are most intense for the first few months following the death, but can persist in varying degrees for years. Mrs WE's expressions of longing, guilt and anger all indicate a normal grieving process.

It is possible that Mrs WE meets the criteria for a complicated grief reaction (Horowitz *et al.* 1997). Ten months after her husband's death, she is still describing anger and bitterness. She also experiences recurrent pangs of painful emotions, with yearnings and longing. To assess this adequately, I should enquire about two further aspects of her bereavement reaction. Is she still expressing a sense of disbelief regarding his death? Does her preoccupation with thoughts of her husband include intrusive distressing thoughts related to his death?

To establish whether Mrs WE might fulfil the criteria for a depressive disorder, I need to enquire about feelings of worthlessness, and any intense feelings of guilt that are not related to the bereavement. I should assess her preoccupation with dying and suicidality, in particular asking about any plans for suicide. I should look for signs of markedly slow speech and movements, and for evidence of prolonged or severe inability to function, such as an inability to socialize or enjoy any leisure activities. Her past history of depression is an indication of increased risk, though there appears to have been only one treated episode, many years ago.

I could follow current guidelines from the NHS Quality and Outcomes Framework, and estimate the severity of her depressive symptoms using a standardized self-rating instrument (BMA and NHS Employers 2006). However this would not help me to distinguish between these three diagnostic categories. Clinical judgement is needed, particularly in deciding what terms like 'intense', 'prolonged' or 'severe' mean in practice. My impression is that there is no convincing evidence from the brief to indicate a depressive disorder in Winifred's case. I think that a complicated grief reaction is the most likely diagnosis.

Social and personal context

I should ask Mrs WE about the level, and quality, of social support that she can access. How strong are her social networks, in particular how much she can rely on family and friends for immediate practical help? This is an important indicator of mental health (Lehtinen 2003). Does she have an active role in relation to family and friends, for example with care of her grandchildren, or within a faith community?

Most importantly, I need to find out what Mrs WE herself wants. My guess would be that she wants two main things: to have her husband back, and to feel safe in her home.

Examination and investigations

It would probably be useful to check her weight and blood pressure, listen to her heart and to enquire – discreetly – about her alcohol intake and smoking habits. Her thyroid function is normal. There is no need for further tests on the basis of this brief, unless she has other problems such as weight loss or excess alcohol intake, in which case I would wish to exclude neoplastic or hepatic pathologies.

Management options

There is little rigorous evidence on which to base recommendations for the best treatment of people experiencing bereavement (Forte *et al.* 2004).

In Mrs WE's case, I can see no good reason to challenge her reluctance to take antidepressant medication. It is probable that she does not fulfil criteria for a major depressive disorder, and NICE Guidelines recommend "watchful waiting" in such cases (NICE 2004a). In any event, meta-analyses of random-ized controlled trials (Walsh *et al.* 2002) and of pharmaceutical evidence presented to the US Food and Drugs Administration (Khan *et al.* 2002, Kirsch *et al.* 2002) suggest that the evidence for efficacy of antidepressants is more equivocal than previously supposed, especially if patients are uncon-vinced about them (Sullivan *et al.* 2003).

Her co-morbid conditions seem stable. I am not convinced of the indica-tions for long-term treatment of previous peptic ulceration in this case, and would consider the possibility of reducing or stopping her lansoprazole.

The main management options are in the *psychological* and *social* spheres: aiming to help her overcome a complicated grief reaction; and ensuring that her social networks are as enabling as possible.

In psychological terms, I think Mrs WE needs help to travel though the (tragically necessary) grieving process, and to begin to look forward again, building up her sense of mastery (Onrust *et al.* 2006) and recreating her personal life goals (Shear *et al.* 2005). As a GP I can give her some of this help myself, but she would probably also benefit from specific psychosocial interventions. This is very much the sort of situation where I tend to look for additional help from the voluntary sector, rather than relying on referral to specialist mental health services.

What should I do?
It is essential that I start by taking Mrs WE's concerns seriously, expressing my sympathy with the pain and distress that she is experiencing. Without this, she is likely to be confirmed in her initial view that there is nothing I can do to help her.

I will tell her about locally available support for people like her. One option is CRUSE, the UK bereavement charity which provides a national helpline and runs local support groups. Another option – which is the one that I will recommend to her – is to take part in a 'Positive Thoughts' course. These courses, derived from group psycho education principles (Dowrick *et al.* 2000), are run regularly in our locality by a voluntary agency: there are specific courses for older people. Sue Martin discusses one such course in the next commentary.

I will follow up the practice nurse's questions, and ask Mrs WE what has been done about the recent spate of burglaries. If need be I will signpost her towards the police, her local councillors or her Member of Parliament. I will also raise the possibility of change of accommodation to a safer environment, for example in sheltered housing, and explain how agencies such as Age Concern can offer advice and guidance.

What next?
I will continue to offer my support to Mrs WE as she goes through the process of grieving, by arranging to see her on a monthly basis.

This will give me the opportunity to review her progress and, if necessary, reconsider the need for formal psychiatric or pharmacological interventions.

My main aim during these subsequent meetings, however, will be to look with Mrs WE for points of *resilience* (Masten 2001), for evidence of her *personal strengths* (Peterson and Seligman 2004). I will ask, for example, if she can remember what she did when things were difficult in the past, or can describe how she overcame a previous serious challenge to herself or to her family. I will discuss her involvement in family and local community life, and over time will encourage her to find new ways of increasing her contribution, and her sense of engagement. In essence, what I will be aiming to do is to help her derive a sense of meaning and purpose (Dowrick 2004): to rediscover herself as someone with skills, abilities and aspirations, as a person able successfully to lead her own life.

Dr Sue Martin, Independent Practitioner and Trainer, Liverpool

The Positive Thoughts course

Hi, I'm Sue and this is my colleague Chris. First of all we'd just like to say how nice it is to see you all here and to thank you for coming to the Positive Thoughts course. We'll introduce ourselves properly in a moment but already there is something very important that we know about the people who have come to this class. You are already positive people. You have all been brave enough to take the chance of coming here because you want some aspect of your life to be different, to be better, for you to feel more in charge. And we can assure you that this course can do that, in different ways for different people. We're not going to say if you do this course everything will be wonderful and you'll never have any problems again. But we will say that you will learn tricks to handle better and more positively what life throws at you. And people who are more positive not only have better mental health, by feeling more content, but also better physical health. There's now evidence that tells us that if we are positive our immune system functions better, or our blood pressure is lower, all things that help keep us feeling well.

So how will this course help to get Mrs WE back to feeling well? As this is a course specifically for older people she is virtually guaranteed to meet someone else there who has experiences similar to her own. They may be at the stage she is, or they may have started to adjust, but they will both understand and accept the reality of where she is and how she feels without too much explanation needed. This in itself is a great relief, that other people, on the surface normal-looking and getting on with their lives, are really just like her.

The course takes a cognitive behavioural approach, based on the assumption that how we think affects how we feel and what we do. But what we have forgotten, or maybe never even worked out, is how we really do feel. How many times when we are asked 'How are you?' do we say 'Fine thanks', without even thinking for a moment how we actually feel. Or we say 'Oh, I've been so busy', which completely bypasses the question of feeling. And if we are to help Mrs WE she needs to both know how she feels and that her feelings are valid.

Each week every participant gets the opportunity to say how they feel in a safe, accepting environment. We do not 'fix' feelings, but acknowledge their validity and explain the importance and value they have in our lives. It is important that each participant understands from the start that this is not a 'therapy' where they just talk, but that they will be required to learn and practise new techniques that will make them feel more positive about their lives. In practice we have found this is a plus for most people, who can, anyway, see no value in 'just talking about my problems over and over again'.

The basic structure and content of each session is a combination of feedback, discussion, relaxation and homework. It is acceptable that the style and manner of presentation may vary. Every week there is homework and one component is always a mood chart, a daily record of how we feel on a score of 1 to 10. This keeps the theme of feelings high on the agenda. Each session lasts approximately two hours. This includes a tea break which further encourages social support among the group. The lecture notes for the instructor are intended to be the basis of the group discussion with the more detailed information being given to the participants in the form of a handout. This means that during the group there is little reading to be done. This bypasses problems with sight and reading skills.

Each week the course has a different theme, for example: (1) How our activities affect our mood; (2) Finding out the things we can do to make ourselves feel better; (3) Some ways to help us change our thoughts. Each theme is developed in the course, both from the taught material but also from the contributions of course members. People are encouraged to bring in material and ideas that have helped them. These are discussed in the course and then there is appropriate homework. The discussions and the social support these generate are important in helping people find their own solutions.

During the course we hope that Mrs WE will come to realize a number of things. First, she will find that many other people have similar problems. Second, she will realize that there are a number of ways of dealing with any given set of circumstances. She is likely to have both given and taken advice over the time of the course. Practical suggestions will have been made to her about how she can lift her mood. Third, her feelings will have been acknowledged, accepted and validated.

Mrs WE will have frequent opportunities to look at her specific difficulties, her grief and her fear of being alone. If she had not already been given practical information we would have provided this, and she would have been signposted to other relevant agencies. A lot of this information would come from within the group.

Some problems do not have easy solutions. Instead we need to learn to live with them, or better still, bypass them. Mrs WE will have learned to generally look after herself better. There are sessions on good eating habits, on rewarding yourself, on letting others help you and on having fun.

Over the eight weeks the course provides many alternative ways of looking at our lives. If Mrs WE can take even one change on board she will feel more in charge of her life. This will herald the start of a belief that her future can improve and she is the one who has the skills to improve it.

Case 3.3 Panic attacks

Mrs Betty C is an 82-year-old retired clerical officer. She has never been treated for anxiety or depression and until 18 months ago was only seen for monitoring of her blood pressure (she has hypertension and takes atenolol and bendrofluazide). She developed polymyalgia rheumatica nine months ago and is still taking a low dose of prednisolone (2 mg daily). For the last four months she has been attending the local Accident and Emergency (A&E) Unit presenting with chest pain and breathlessness and has been ringing the practice once or twice a week asking to speak to the GP. This behaviour has escalated over the past two months and her own GP is trying to manage her by seeing her weekly, in order to avoid what seemed to be almost daily phone calls. The other GPs in the practice are becoming frustrated by the repeated requests for telephone advice, and by the letters from A&E which request that Mrs BC should be reviewed, as well as the repeated short-term prescriptions for benzodiazepines which are being given by A&E junior staff.

Mrs BC's son, who lives at some distance, has left a message saying that his mother has always been anxious, but it is now getting out of hand and she is ringing him twice and three times a day. He does not feel that he can manage the situation for much longer.

Mrs BC attends the GP presenting as an emergency at the desk and very agitated and tells the GP she cannot go on with these feelings. She described constant 'butterflies' in her stomach and a feeling of nausea and shortness of breath. She can't sleep as she is aware of her heart beating very fast. She has stopped going to her lunch club and had to run out of church on Sunday because she felt so awful.

How can the GP manage this lady's frequent presentations to the practice and to A&E? What might a psychologist offer? How should the son's concerns be addressed?

Dr Ruth Thompson, General Practitioner, Manchester
Mrs BC has presented today in crisis. Her symptoms have been brewing for over a year but the GP should resist any feelings that this is not an emergency. Often patients only seek help when their symptoms become so distressing or interfere so profoundly with their lifestyle that they are willing to contemplate

a change. So, hoping that no other patients with similar emergencies arrive, I ask Mrs BC into my consulting room.

If she is very distressed she may be hyperventilating. This provides an opportunity to talk Mrs BC through behavioural techniques to control breathing 'big breath out, breathe in, hold it 1, 2, 3, breathe out'. Once she is calm she can start to tell her story. As she describes her symptoms I would focus on those that may have pathological causes (for example dyspnoea caused by chronic obstructive pulmonary disease, anaemia or heart failure or palpitations caused thyrotoxicosis or cardiac arrhythmias). A thorough history, including time of day of presentation, duration, severity and associated symptoms, may point to other pathology. Similarly depression and psychosis may both present with anxiety symptoms. As 'anxiety' is essentially a diagnosis of exclusion, the GP's first job must be to exclude other pathology and in an elderly patient this may be quite time-consuming, although this should not be considered as time wasted. The time spent on the initial physical examination, subsequent blood tests and other investigations will provide opportunity to build rapport and to elicit any concerns the patient may have about her symptoms. Specific concerns may result from events such as witnessing a friend presenting with a similar set of symptoms who then went on to develop serious pathology. Though obviously I would weigh up the risk involved in medical investigation and reinforcing her health anxiety, I may need to refer her for a physical investigation that will address her concerns. She may need a referral to a secondary care consultant and the letter would have to outline that I am considering a diagnosis of anxiety and be specific about my aims for the referral. It may be virtually impossible to move towards a diagnosis of anxiety, without excluding specific pathology. If she seems to have a fixed belief that she has a physical problem as a cause for her symptoms, it may not be helpful to discuss anxiety or mental health issues at this appointment. It is important to reassure Mrs BC that the expectation is that most of the tests will be normal, and that I believe her symptoms to be treatable and that I will be responsible for her follow-up.

In this initial appointment it is also necessary to cover risk assessment. Mrs BC's symptoms may be a presentation of a depressive illness. If so her symptoms may have become so distressing to her that she has contemplated harming herself. By suggesting that other people in her situation have feelings of harm she may disclose suicidal ideation. If this is the case I may need to consider referring her either to the on-call psychiatrist or for an urgent assessment by an old-age psychiatrist. If she is not expressing feelings or thoughts that she would harm herself, I would explore more fully for any symptoms of depression, asking her about her mood, her concentration, her appetite and weight and whether she can distract herself from her panic or her low mood to enjoy anything.

I would attempt to negotiate with her some setting of boundaries. Her usual GP may be willing to hand her over for a period of time and it would be important for her to have an appointment made for a weekly consultation. The practice reception staff all need to know that she has a weekly appointment. Ideally if she phones the practice prior to attending and if she is breathless, it may be necessary for the GP or triage nurse to do breathing instructions over the phone and then reassure her that she can wait until her weekly appointment. It is impossible to prevent attendances at the A&E department, and it would be bad practice to do so, although it is vital to discuss with Mrs BC her reasons for attending and her expectations from attending A&E. The NICE Guidelines on anxiety (NICE 2004b) have a section written for A&E departments. After discussion with the local A&E and out-of-hours service it may be possible to limit the benzodiazepine prescriptions. Not setting and working within suitable boundaries is one of the major barriers to successful intervention.

As the results of the tests prove to be normal, we would then broach the issue of a diagnosis of anxiety and depression. It may be useful to present anxiety in terms of a maladaptive flight/fight response which results in excessive adrenaline production and causes the symptoms. Depression can be presented as lack of enjoyment and inability to enjoy things, or by reflecting her own symptoms back to her. Alternatively I might run through a schedule such as PHQ-9 or the GDS-15 (see Chapter 7) and reflect a high score back to her, suggesting that she may have a depressive illness.

It may be that she is resistant to a diagnosis of a mental health problem, and if her anxiety symptoms are predominant, with physical symptoms and worries, the reattribution model (Morriss and Gask 2002) may be useful. The aim of reattribution is to normalize the patient's interpretations of their bodily symptoms, modify their beliefs about causes of their symptoms, and treat any underlying depression. Challenging Mrs BC's beliefs that there is a physical cause for the symptoms can move her towards an acceptance that symptoms may have a psychological component. Ideally, with Mrs BC's consent, her son would be invited to attend to subsequent appointments. If he accepts 'anxiety' or 'depression' as a possible diagnosis he may be able to play a role in challenging Mrs BC if she has a fixed belief in a physical cause. Throughout, I would need to monitor her physical symptoms and, if changing, we would have to revisit the original diagnosis.

Once anxiety, with or without depressive symptoms, has been diagnosed and the diagnosis accepted by the patient, we can move forward with different treatment options. The NICE Guidelines on anxiety (NICE 2004b) recommend using a cognitive behavioural therapy (CBT) model and this can either be delivered by a suitably trained GP, community mental health worker or a psychologist, or be self-directed using the Internet (the mood gym), self-help leaflets or books. Mike Morley (see next section) discusses how CBT may be applied to Mrs BC's case. The change in church and luncheon club attendance is one aspect of behaviour that may be important. A random act of violence, being mugged for example, may have left her feeling vulnerable. If this has happened she may have got trapped in a vicious circle of negative behaviour, in which anxiety symptoms on leaving the house have led to worry about collapsing or embarrassing herself in public which in turn stops her going out, in turn reinforcing the feelings of anxiety. A short course of CBT may help her to recognize the behaviours and the beliefs that are perpetuating the anxiety symptoms. Using breathing techniques as the main way of preventing the physical symptoms of adrenaline, she may be able to challenge the beliefs and alter the behaviour that perpetuate the anxiety. The ability of the patient to benefit from CBT is dependent on their ability to understand and accept the disease model presented to them and their part in altering it. It is often difficult to obtain CBT at a time of crisis, but GPs can learn basic techniques to use whilst patients wait for an appointment with a counsellor or psychologist. It is also useful to find out what resources are available locally using the voluntary sector.

Some patients and doctors just want an immediate cessation of symptoms which is why this patient has been prescribed several courses of benzodiazepines in the past. Though benzodiazepines are effective in reducing symptoms of anxiety in the short term, they have serious consequences of dependence in the long term. This is the rationale behind NICE guidance for generalized anxiety disorder: 'benzodiazepines should not usually be used beyond 2–4 weeks' (NICE 2004b). In an older patient there is the concern of sedation and associated with increased risk of falls (Sorock and Shimkin 1988). Pharmacological options that could be offered would include beta-blockers which could be offered short term for management of symptoms of anxiety and may enable Mrs BC to embark on CBT. In an elderly patient it is important to have a normal electrocardiogram (ECG) and thorough check for asthma prior to starting them. Other pharmacological interventions may include antidepressants either selective serotonin reuptake inhibitors (SSRIs) or a tricyclic antidepressant (TCA) such as imipramine, although the side effects, drug interactions and risk in overdose make me less likely to prescribe TCAs. If Mrs BC has significant and persistent depressive symptoms, with a PHQ-9 supporting a diagnosis of depression, then I would encourage her to try antidepressants. The NICE (2004a) guidance suggests that if a patient still has significant symptoms after two interventions (which include psychological or pharmacological) then they should be referred to specialist mental health services. The possibility of referral depends on local organization of services, but I would try to speak to an old-age psychiatrist for advice and refer the patient if the patient was willing to attend and the local referral guidelines permitted this.

Dr Michael Morley, Consultant Clinical Psychologist, Manchester Mental Health and Social Care Trust
In principle all evidence-based psychological therapies available to younger adults for depression should also be available to older adults (NICE 2004a,

2004b). However in resource-limited services the framework of a stepped care approach is appropriate. Bower and Gilbody (2005) suggest there are probably four qualitatively different steps in psychological therapies: pure self-help (no therapist input beyond assessment); guided self-help and group therapy (therapist input around 1–2 hours per patient); brief individual therapy (therapist input around 6 hours per patient); and longer-term individual therapy (therapist input around 16 hours per patient).

In the UK clinical psychologists are trained in a broad range of psychological assessments and evidence-based psychological therapies, and can work as lone practitioners or in multidisciplinary teams. A comprehensive reassessment in close collaboration with the GP would allow a care plan to be developed that could offer Mrs BC a choice of pharmacological and/or psychological treatments for depression and anxiety. The prescribing and monitoring of anti-depressants should be undertaken by the GP, the psychological intervention would be undertaken by the clinical psychologist; co-ordination of the treatment and its effectiveness might be monitored jointly.

As mentioned by Ruth Thompson (see previous section), scientific review and recent policy guidance predominantly identify cognitive behavioural therapy (CBT) as the front-line psychological treatment but there is merit in also considering other therapies when working with older people, such as inter-personal therapy (Klerman *et al.* 1984) and systemic therapy (Jones and Asen 1999). However, here I will apply CBT principles to Mrs BC's case.

An initial interview with Mrs BC by the clinical psychologist to gather general information needs to be supplemented by a more specific psychological therapy interview, to assess her overall suitability for a particular approach, and derive a treatment plan. The general assessment of an older adult has already been outlined and would include at least a comprehensive review of physical, psychological and social needs, a fuller description of treatments thus far tried and a risk assessment. Information should also be collected about current circumstances which might include living conditions, risk of isolation, and quality of inter-personal relationships. The process of helping an individual define what might need to change in relation to the therapy is very often a work in progress in the early stages of therapy, but a thorough assessment will offer clear pointers in the first instance.

CBT refers to a structured therapy which broadly covers a range of behavioural and cognitive therapy models. In brief, behavioural models of depression suggest that the general reduction in levels of activity associated with a reduced frequency of social reinforcement (for example avoiding lunch club and church) are potential mechanisms in maintaining depression (Lewinsohn 1975). CBT models of depression emphasize that the content and style of a person's thinking become more negative and biased when they are depressed (Beck *et al.* 1979). When an individual like Mrs BC is depressed their thinking is characterized by themes of loss, vulnerability, failure and defeat. Some people who are not depressed have pre-existing unhelpful beliefs that make them more prone to depression, especially in the face of adverse circumstances. An example in Mrs BC's case might be recent health difficulties triggering health-related fears. In addition, other cognitive models suggest that individuals who are anxious focus their attention in specific ways on what they perceive to be threatening. Individual appraisal of supposed threat and danger is biased leading them to overestimate the likely occurrence of an event (e.g. 'these feelings are awful', 'something must be wrong', 'I need help now') and underestimate how they will cope, without additional help. The anxious individual thus engages in various 'safety behaviours' (telephoning GP and/ or son, attendance at GP surgery or A&E department) designed to lower anxiety and stay safe, but more often these behaviours usually sustain the biased thinking, which reinforces the anxiety.

A psychological therapy is not something to be done to an individual but very much relies on building a shared view/conceptualization of the difficulties, within a strong therapeutic alliance. For example, CBT is fundamentally about helping an individual understand and alter their emotional response(s), and is not about reducing a person's beliefs and behaviour to a formulaic set of frequencies of reinforcement or patterns of irrational thinking. The emphasis is on normalizing the often frightening and bewildering symptoms of anxiety and depression, and on emphasizing that though distressing the symptoms can be viewed as understandable reactions to particular situations and life events. The range of older adult experience should prompt caution in arriving at a case conceptualization 'too early', without adequate information. Information from both the general and CBT-specific interview would seek to understand Mrs BC's formative experiences especially her (core) beliefs about interpersonal and social interactions, health and ill health, as well as family and support networks (Laidlaw et al. 2003). In this way valuable information can be gained to help guide the CBT treatment plan, and also understand the patient more fully.

Thus, a broad-based CBT approach would involve identifying an individual's current needs and developing cognitive and or behavioural interventions to help with current stressors. This involves teaching patients to be more aware of negative bias in their thinking, whether long-standing or in response to current difficulties, and to discover more helpful patterns of thinking and behaving. Individuals are taught to view their thoughts and beliefs as testable hypotheses and encouraged to take graded risks in confronting feared situations in order to disconfirm their predictions, and reduce safety behaviours. The approach is structured by the psychologist to help the person (and significant others, such as the son, in this case) orient to behavioural and cognitive tasks within and across sessions. Supplementary written information about psychological models of depression are important adjuncts in the normalizing process, as well as helping to identify stages of therapy, including producing a blueprint for relapse. The individual is taught to recognize mood fluctuations and vulnerabilities, to develop strategies that enhance coping abilities, reduce avoidant behaviours, increase activities, and also learn to manage and accept certain feelings in difficult situations.

Editors' comments

We feel that the following points are particularly important in the first three cases.

Notes on Case 3.1

- Requests for sleeping tablets should alert the GP to the possibility of a mental health problem, but adequate history-taking to exclude an organic disease or side effects of drugs is needed.
- Careful observation and an open consultation style are important in uncovering undisclosed depression in later life.
- Screening questions for depression are a useful way for the health-care professionals to explore mood.
- In this scenario of mild depression 'watchful waiting' with arrangement for structured follow-up is emphasized, but this does not mean 'do nothing' – sleep hygiene, behavioural activation and social contact are important in this case as is the role of 'signposting' to appropriate sources of help.
- Step 1 of the stepped care approach involves a co-ordinated approach from primary care team members.

Notes on Case 3.2

- Differentiation of grief from depression involves an exploration of biological symptoms of depression, finding out about a previous history of a mood disorder and assessment of risk of self-harm.
- It is important to find out what the patient wants and assess their attitudes to medication.
- GPs can offer simple psychotherapeutic interventions to help the grieving process.
- Interventions based on cognitive behavioural or problem-solving principles are often available in the voluntary sector and health-care professionals should make themselves aware of local agencies which can help.
- The case also illustrates the therapeutic potential of helping older people in a group setting. This can also counter the social withdrawal often seen in late-life depression.

Notes on Case 3.3

- Anxiety often coexists with depression, and may be the predominant symptom.
- Setting boundaries can be a useful way of containing acute presentations and providing feedback to patients that they can, in fact, manage their symptoms.
- CBT is useful for mixed anxiety and depression: it relies on therapist and patient developing a shared view of the difficulties and helping the person to understand their emotional responses.
- Although minor modifications may be needed to address sensory impairment, etc., CBT does not require any major modifications to the model when used with older people.
- Referral to a higher step may be required to access psychological interventions.
- Anxiolytic drugs have a very limited role in anxious depression and should only be used short term.

The next chapter deals with more complicated cases of late-life depression.

REFERENCES

Audit Commission (1999) *First Assessment: A Review of District Nursing in England and Wales.* London: Audit Commission.

Banerjee S., Shamash K., Macdonald A. J. D., Mann A. H. (1996) Randomized controlled trial of effect of intervention by psychogeriatric team on depression in frail elderly people at home. *Br. Med. J.* **313**, 1058–61.

Beck A. T., Rush A. J., Shaw B. F., *et al.* (1979) *Cognitive Therapy of Depression.* New York: John Wiley.

BMA and NHS Employers (2006) *Revisions to the GMS Contract, 2006/7: Delivering Investment in General Practice.* London: British Medical Association.

Bower P., Gilbody S. (2005) Stepped care in psychological therapies: access, effectiveness and efficiency: narrative literature review. *Br. J. Psychiatry* **186**, 11–17.

Burroughs H., Morley M., Lovell K., *et al.* (2006) 'Justifiable depression': how health professionals and patients view late-life depression – a qualitative study. *Fam. Practice* **23**, 369–77.

D'Ath P., Katona P., Mullan E., Evans S., Katona C. (1994) Screening, detection and management of depression in elderly primary care attendees: the acceptability and performance of the 15-item geriatric Depression Scale (GDS15) and the development of short versions. *Fam. Practice* **11**, 260–6.

Department of Health (2001) *National Service Framework for Older People.* London: HMSO.

Department of Health (2006) *Improving Access to Psychological Therapies.* London: The Stationery Office.

Dowrick C. (2004) *Beyond Depression: A New Approach to Understanding and Management.* Oxford, UK: Oxford University Press.

Dowrick C., Dunn G., Dalgard O. S., *et al.* (2000) Problem-solving treatment and group psycho-education for depression: a multicentre randomized controlled trial. *Br. Med. J.* **321**, 1450–4.

Forte A. L., Hill M., Pazder R., *et al.* (2004) Bereavement care interventions: a systematic review. *Biomed. Centr. Palliat. Care* **3**, 3.

Horowitz M. J., Siegel B., Holen A., *et al.* (1997) Diagnostic criteria for complicated grief disorder. *Am. J. Psychiatry* **174**, 67–73.

Jones E., Asen E. (1999) *Systemic Couple Therapy and Depression.* London: Karnac.

Katona C., Freeling P., Hinchcliffe K. (1995). Recognition and management of depression in late life in general practice: consensus statement. *Prim. Care Psychiatry* **1**, 107–13.

Khan A., Khan S., Brown W. A. (2002) Are placebo controls necessary to test new antidepressants and anxiolytics? *Int. J. Neuropsychopharmacol.* **3**, 193–7.

Kirsch I., Moore T. J., Scoboria A., *et al.* (2002) The Emperor's New Drugs: an analysis of antidepressant medication data submitted to the US Food and Drug Administration. *Prevention and Treatment* **5**, Article 23.

Klerman G. L., Weissman M. M. Rounsaville B. J., *et al.* (1984) *Interpersonal Psychotherapy of Depression.* New York: Basic Books.

Laidlaw K., Thompson L. W., Dick-Sisin L., Gallagher-Thompson D. (2003) *Cognitive Behaviour Therapy with Older People.* Chichester, UK: John Wiley.

Lehtinen V., Michalak E., Wilkinson C., *et al.* (2003) Urban–rural differences in the occurrence of depressive disorder in Europe: evidence from the ODIN study. *Soc. Psychiatry Psychiatr. Epidemiol.* **38**, 283–9.

Lewinsohn P. M. (1975) The behavioral study and treatment of depression. In *Progress in Behavior Modification*, vol. 1, eds. M. Hersen, R. M. Eisler and P. M. Miller. New York: Academic Press, pp. 19–64.

Masten A. S. (2001) Ordinary magic: resilience processes in development. *Am. Psychol.* **56**, 227–38.

Morriss R. K., Gask L. (2002) Treatment of patients with somatized mental disorder: effects of reattribution training on outcomes under the direct control of the family doctor. *Psychosomatics* **43**, 394–9.

Murray Parkes C. (1998) *Bereavement: Studies of Grief in Adult Life*, 3rd edn. London: Routledge/Psychology Press.

NICE (2004a) *Depression: Management of Depression in Primary and Secondary Care*, Clinical Guideline No. 23. London: National Institute for Health and Clinical Excellence.

NICE (2004b). *Anxiety: Management of Anxiety in Adults in Primary, Secondary and Community care*, Clinical Guideline NO. 22. London: National Institute for Health and Clinical Excellence.

Onrust S., Cuijpers P., Smit F., *et al.* (2006) Predictors of psychological adjustment after bereavement. *Int. Psychogeriatrics* **14**, 1–15.

Peterson C., Seligman M. (2004) *Character Strengths and Virtues: A Handbook and Classification.* Washington, DC: American Psychological Association.

Shear K., Frank E., Houck P. R., Reynolds C. F. (2005) Treatment of complicated grief: a randomized controlled trial. *J. Am. Med. Assoc.* **293**, 2601–8.

Shiekh J., Yesavage J. (1986) Geriatric Depression Scale: recent findings and development of a short version. In *Clinical Gerontology: A Guide to Assessment and Intervention*, ed. T. Brink. New York: Howarth Press, pp. 165–75.

Sorock G. S., Shimkin E. E. (1988) Benzodiazepine sedatives and the risk of falling in a community-dwelling elderly cohort. *Arch. Intern. Med.* **148**, 2441–4.

Sullivan M., Katon W., Russo J., *et al.* (2003) Patients' beliefs predict response to paroxetine among primary care patients with dysthymia and minor depression. *J. Am. Board Fam. Pract.* **16**, 22–31.

Walsh B. T., Seidman S. N., Sysko R., *et al.* (2002) Placebo response in studies of major depression. *J. Am. Med. Assoc.* **287**, 1840–7.

4

Management of more complicated depression in primary care: case studies UK

The next commentaries illustrate the management of patients with increasingly complex problems where the management needs to be integrated with other professionals.

Case 4.1 Hidden alcohol consumption

Mrs Ruth M is a 79-year-old lady who attends the practice infrequently, only when she needs her blood checking for thyroid function (she has been on thyroxine for 10 years) and her flu vaccine with the practice nurse. She makes an appointment with her GP as she has been feeling really run down recently and wonders if the dose of thyroxine needs changing. She is having difficulty sleeping and has tended to withdraw from her usual activities (going to the library and reading, meeting her friends for a drink in their local pub). She admits to the GP that she does 'enjoy a tipple' and feels that she might have been drinking more than usual in the past few months. She often has a drink with her mid-morning coffee as it stops her feeling so awful, and she has always had a couple of whiskies in the evening to help her sleep, but that doesn't seem to be working at the moment.

What factors should be taken into account in the assessment of this patient's mood?

How should Mrs RM be investigated?

Who might the GP work with in the management of this patient?

Dr Elizabeth Murray, General Practitioner and Reader in Primary Care, Royal Free and University College Medical School, London, and James Oliver, Substance Abuse Counsellor, Lonsdale Medical Centre, London

Assessment

Background

Mrs RM has probably found it difficult to admit to feeling low and run down, and is likely to have delayed coming to the doctor. She is an infrequent

Integrated Management of Depression in the Elderly, ed. C. Chew-Graham, R. Baldwin and A. Burns. Published by Cambridge University Press. © Cambridge University Press 2008.

attender, which suggests she avoids 'bothering' the doctor, and is frightened of 'wasting the doctor's time'. This generation of patients may be still very appreciative of the National Health Service, and have often survived very difficult times, either in the Great Depression of the 1930s, in the Second World War, or subsequently during the lean years of the 1950s. As a result of these experiences, she may have a relatively stoic approach to life, and a high threshold for admitting distress. Hence her approach to the doctor needs to be taken seriously, with the doctor moving fairly swiftly to active assessment and intervention, rather than taking the 'wait and see' approach that can be appropriate with more frequent attenders.

Alcohol misuse and depression often coexist (Devanand 2002, Pettinati 2004) and it can be hard to disentangle which came first. Continued alcohol misuse tends to prolong depression and inhibits recovery, while continued depression worsens the prognosis for recovery from alcohol misuse. From a general practice perspective, it is probably better to address both problems simultaneously, rather than wondering which came first.

The aim of the assessment

Mrs RM has two problems (also called a 'dual diagnosis') – she appears to be depressed, and she appears to misuse alcohol. The aim of the assessment is to determine the severity of both problems, so that appropriate treatment can be instituted. Her depression may be mild, moderate or severe. She may be drinking excessively or hazardously, or she may be dependent on alcohol.

Three types of elderly drinkers have been identified:
(1) Early-onset drinkers or 'survivors'. These are people who have a continuing problem with alcohol which developed in earlier life. It is thought that about two-thirds of elderly problem drinkers have had an early onset of alcohol misuse.
(2) Late onset drinkers or 'reactors'. These begin problematic drinking later in life, often in response to life events (bereavement, loneliness, retirement, pain, insomnia).
(3) Intermittent or 'binge' drinkers who use alcohol occasionally but to excess. Both 'reactors' and 'binge' drinkers have a high chance of managing their alcohol problem with adequate treatment and support (Institute of Alcohol Studies 1999).

Assessment of depression

The assessment of depression has been well covered elsewhere in this book. The important features to cover here include Mrs RM's views about the problem, including her views on the cause, any triggers for depression, her level of social support, and her physical health, including pain, insomnia, mobility, hearing and vision, and what she has already tried to help herself get better.

It is important to undertake an assessment of the severity of her depression to determine whether she has mild, moderate or severe depression, as treatment varies according to level of severity. The PHQ-9 (Patient Health Questionnaire – see Chapter 7) can be particularly useful (Kroenke, *et al.* 2001). This is a self-completion questionnaire, and the scoring system classifies respondents as mildly, moderately or severely depressed.

Assessment of the alcohol problem

The main information needed to assess Mrs RM's alcohol problem include:

- how much she is drinking
- level of dependency
- reasons for drinking
- current beliefs about the effect of alcohol on her health, and level of motivation for reducing alcohol intake.

The best way of estimating Mrs RM's alcohol intake is to take a formal alcohol history. This involves asking her about the amount drunk on each of the last seven days, starting with the most recent day, and working back. For each day, enquire whether she had anything to drink at all that day. If yes, work through the day (evening, afternoon, lunch, morning) to get a report of what alcohol she drank, and how much of it.

This can then be translated into units, using the formula:

$$(\text{amount drunk in ml} \times \%\text{ABV [alcohol by volume]})/1000.$$

The guidelines for safe drinking in younger adults are 14 units per week for women and 21 units per week for men. However, older people are more sensitive to harm from alcohol, as they metabolize alcohol less efficiently, and their brain is more affected. Hence the guidelines for safe drinking in older people are no more than one drink per day for men or women (Blow 2000).

Data from the USA suggest that although about 12% of older women misuse alcohol, fewer than 1% are dependent (Blow 2000). Dependency can be assessed from asking whether she drinks every day, when she has her first drink in the day, and what happens if she does not have it. If she has a significant level of dependency, indicated by physical withdrawal symptoms if she delays taking alcohol, she should not try to stop drinking suddenly without adequate medical help and medication cover, as this is dangerous and potentially life-threatening.

It is important to find out why Mrs RM is drinking, and what she thinks it does for her health. If she is drinking to self-medicate for pain or insomnia, part of the treatment plan will involve finding alternative solutions to these problems. Knowing her current level of motivation for addressing her alcohol problem will help target appropriate advice and information.

Assessment of physical health

Alcohol affects almost every organ in the body, and many people who drink excessively have other behaviours that may pose a risk to their health, such as smoking, eating a poor diet and avoiding exercise. It is worth checking on these, and important to ask about diet, as Mrs RM may be developing sub-clinical malnutrition.

The GP will need to check her blood pressure (alcohol is cardiotoxic and can raise blood pressure), her weight (to confirm a clinical impression of whether she is obese from the excess calories in alcohol, or malnourished from neglect), and check her urine for sugar (as alcohol can precipitate diabetes). Other physical examination will be guided by the doctor's initial assessment – if she appears unwell, the GP should examine her more thoroughly than if she appears well, particularly being aware of cardiomegaly (as alcohol can cause cardiomyopathy), hepatomegaly (from liver damage) and neuropathy.

Baseline investigations should include a full blood count (she may have anaemia due to occult blood loss from gastritis, or a macrocytosis from her alcohol intake), liver function tests (including the gamma-globulin test – the most sensitive marker for alcohol-related liver damage), and thyroid function tests (as she thinks her low mood is related to her thyroid). Her fasting lipids are very likely to be elevated in view of her alcohol intake, and her glucose may be abnormal. Any follow-up investigations will be determined by the initial results – for example, if Mrs RM has a palpable liver with abnormal liver function tests she will need a liver ultrasound.

Treatment

Treatment depends on the results of the assessment, and needs to address both Mrs RM's problems: depression and alcohol misuse. Management begins as soon as Mrs RM presents to the GP – praise for attending, recognition and naming of the problems, and reassurance that these are treatable problems which are likely to get better are all important early therapeutic interventions. The research evidence supports the integration of mental health and substance abuse services for clients with dual diagnoses (Sacks 2000); unfortunately this is not common practice in the UK.

Treatment of depression

If Mrs RM is not dependent on alcohol, it is well worth explaining to her that her alcohol intake is contributing to her depression. If she stops drinking she is very likely to feel less depressed within a few weeks.

The use of antidepressants in people with dual diagnoses (depression and alcohol misuse) can be controversial. Some people argue that as alcohol is a depressant, there is little point treating depression until the patient has stopped drinking. However, the evidence supports active treatment of both problems (alcohol and depression) (Sullivan *et al*. 2005). Antidepressants help lift mood, while additional interventions are needed for the alcohol problem.

NICE Guidelines confirm that older adults benefit as much as younger people from treatment for depression (NICE 2004). Selective serotonin reuptake inhibitors (SSRIs) such as fluoxetine or citalopram are particularly suitable for use in someone with coexisting alcohol problems, as they are relatively safe in overdose. As SSRIs can cause agitation and temporary worsening of symptoms, people do need review one to two weeks after starting medication, and less frequently thereafter until stabilized.

Treatment for alcohol problems

If Mrs RM is not physically dependent on alcohol, she can be well managed in primary care. Ideally she should be supported by her GP, and a professional adequately trained in psychological support or counselling people with coexisting mental health and substance misuse problems. Unfortunately recent evidence suggests only one in 18 people who need help for alcohol problems receive it (Drummond *et al*. 2004), and not all community alcohol workers are adequately trained to respond appropriately to people with dual diagnoses. Hence the GP will need to check the level of expertise of the community alcohol worker, and, if the worker is not highly trained, may need to provide additional support, or seek support from the old-age mental health services.

There is a strong evidence base for brief interventions in hazardous or excessive drinkers (Moyer *et al*. 2002). Simply calculating the total weekly alcohol intake and reflecting that back to the patient often triggers change, particularly if coupled with simple health information about the harms of alcohol. If the GP does not have access to a community alcohol worker such a brief intervention coupled with supportive monitoring and review is likely to benefit Mrs RM.

A well-trained alcohol counsellor is likely to use motivational enhancement therapy (or motivational interviewing) and/or cognitive behavioural therapy (CBT). Both these approaches have a strong evidence base. Motivational enhancement therapy aims to move people into a position where they will consider change, while CBT looks at a person's thoughts and beliefs, and how these interact with drinking behaviour. As has been discussed by Mike Morley (see Case 3.3, in the previous chapter), CBT is effective in treating older people with depression (Scogin and McElreath 1994), and addressing the negative beliefs typical of depression is an important part of the CBT work in substance abuse (Beck *et al*. 1993).

She will need a great deal of support both while reducing or stopping alcohol, but also in the weeks and months after. People often have 'slips', and these need careful handling. There is a risk that after a 'slip' the person will feel guilty and suffer from low self-esteem, and that these feelings of worthlessness will result in renewed alcohol intake. Part of the support needed is reassurance that 'slips' are a normal part of recovery, and that what is important is learning from each slip, and working out how to deal with future similar situations without recourse to alcohol.

Addressing underlying factors
If the factors that led Mrs RM to drink excessively are not addressed, there is a high chance that she will relapse. A referral to social services may help, if there are financial problems, problems with social isolation, or difficulties with activities of daily living. Alternatively a local voluntary organization may be able to assist with befriending or practical help.

In the longer term
Mrs RM has a good prognosis, and is likely to make a good recovery. However, she does remain at increased risk for both depression and alcohol misuse and will need to be kept under regular review by the GP.

Case 4.2 Physical co-morbidity

Mr Wasif H has diabetes and hypertension and until his retirement six months ago, he had managed both conditions effectively. He had worked as a lecturer in engineering at a local college, but had been asked to retire fully at the age of 65 years, and had found the transition very difficult. He consulted his GP complaining of worsening pain in his left hip and both knees and admitting that he had stopped going out unless his wife drove him, and was spending long periods just sitting at home 'looking at the world going by'. His conversations at home seem increasingly to do with how badly his life has turned out, wondering what he has done 'to deserve this endless pain'. He now worries constantly about his diabetes and blood pressure, but admits forgetting to take his tablets (ramipril, gliclazide, atorvastatin and aspirin) and being rather lax with his diet for the past couple of months. He worries that he might have a heart attack, like his father, and that his painful joints would mean he would soon be confined to a wheelchair. He had been taken to A&E at the local hospital by his son twice in the past month complaining once of hip pain, and once because he had not taken his tablets for two days, and his family were finding it difficult to cope with his inactivity. His son comments that his father was previously a proud man who achieved well professionally after coming to England in the 1960s, and who had been ambitious for his family. He now seems to be uninterested in his family, preferring to be on his own.

Discuss the assessment and management of Mr WH. How could his pain be managed?

Dr Avril Danczak, General Practitioner and GP Tutor and Trainer, Manchester Primary Care Trust

Assessment

Assessment of Mr WH should include physical, psychological, social and 'existential or spiritual' considerations.

Assessment for physical disease will include an appropriate examination to exclude possible underlying physical causes for his joint problems (e.g. vitamin D deficiency, arthritis, secondaries from cancer, etc.) and ensuring that his diabetes and hypertension medications are appropriate, checking for side effects and assessing treatment concordance. Investigations (full blood count, inflammatory markers such as erythrocyte sedimentation rate and C-reactive protein) may be needed if clinical examination suggests a more sinister cause for his pain. In addition, assessment of renal and thyroid function and monitoring of diabetes should be considered.

Psychological assessment of mood, sleep, motivation, concentration and enjoyment of activities needs tact and perhaps a longer consultation, inviting the patient back in the next few days if this cannot be achieved today. With his permission, involving the family in this assessment (for example the son) may be very illuminating and may also result in gaining allies within the family, to support him in enacting a management plan. It may be necessary to see the father and son together and separately. The risk of self-harm and suicide needs to be clarified by exploring whether Mr WH has any plans for the future, has thought about harming himself and, if he has, why does he not act on these thoughts.

His social context needs to be understood. Sometimes the family circumstances are already well known to the GP. Understanding relationships at home, who is there to support him and what activities he may be able to engage in, will aid sensible management planning. Knowing family members and their views may avoid misunderstandings in the delivery of care.

Management

The different components of his distress need to be openly acknowledged. His change of life circumstances, chronic illness and current inactivity all promote low mood and make the experience of pain worse. This process should be articulated clearly to ensure that a holistic approach is explicit and recognized by all parties. This avoids the futile 'it's not in my mind, doctor' conversation with the patient.

Discussion and ventilation of thoughts and feelings is crucial. Use of medication such as antidepressants needs discussion with the patient, and possibly with family members, including a sensitive exploration of the acceptability and purposes of medication, possible duration of treatment and other concerns that may surface such as a fear of addiction.

Explore with Mr WH why he thinks his life has turned out badly when others might see him as being successful. What were his expectations on coming to Britain? Have these been met? Was his retirement handled tactfully or carelessly? What other losses of role or of social support has he experienced which might relate to his present mood disorder? What are his main concerns and his fears for the future? Can these be addressed?

Co-morbidities and optimizing management of physical conditions must be fully addressed.

If discussion with me over a series of consultations with or without medication does not work then increased involvement by other teams may be helpful (NICE 2004).

Psychological interventions could include a recommendation to increase activity, and 'exercise on prescription' (an NHS initiative in primary care designed to increase activity and mobility in groups at risk of conditions such as coronary artery disease, osteoporosis or those with depression) or to the primary mental care team (who provide support, self-help or problem-solving approaches to people with mild to moderate mental health problems). GPs can use their local knowledge to access community voluntary and statutory services such as day centres, cultural groups (e.g. a group for African-Caribbeans, Indian Senior Citizens Association, etc.) and these should be used to the full.

Regular follow-up by the GP will mean continued discussion of the issues concerning the patient, and review of the effectiveness of interventions the patient chooses. Using screening tools (such as the PHQ – see Chapter 7) may create an over-medicalized approach to an already complex situation but can be a useful adjunct to a review of effectiveness or aid in the decision of whether to prescribe antidepressants.

Collaboration between primary and secondary care

If improvement is still delayed or incomplete, discussion about the management of the patient with a psychiatrist may result in helpful suggestions. This may forestall a referral which some patients find stigmatizing. However, referral for further assessment is warranted if primary care management fails or the GP feels the patient is at real risk of self-harm or self-neglect (NICE 2004).

Barriers to effective management

This patient seems to have a somatized form of depression and may be unwilling to think about psychological or psychiatric explanations for his feelings or for his pain. His family may or may not agree with the formulation and families are often anxious about physical disease. This will need careful handling in the discussion and an explicit acknowledgement that both physical and psychological issues can be managed simultaneously. A proud man with a prominent position in his local community may be less willing to access services, particularly those aimed at people with mental health problems. Specific suggestions that are appropriate to him may have to be developed. If this approach does not work he might benefit from CBT, although availability of CBT, particularly for the elderly, can be quite restricted in the UK.

Managing his pain will need a combined approach, including psychological and physical intervention such as advising continued activity, prescription of calcium and vitamin D supplements if appropriate, ensuring adequate analgesia and considering the use of antidepressants. It is sometimes helpful to frame the use of antidepressants as being of benefit as an adjunct to pain relief rather than primarily for the management of psychological symptoms. This may make their use more acceptable to the patient and the family.

This man has experienced a profound but unacknowledged alteration of his social role following retirement which may make a 'medical' approach seem more acceptable to him. Open discussion may help and he may even benefit from referral to retirement planning classes such as are available locally via the Citizens' Advice Bureau. He could be encouraged to become more active in helping other members of his community and thus regain a role in his culture and context.

Summary

To manage this patient effectively requires him to be seen in the round, not merely as an example of a 'somatized depression' but as a human being who has experienced success, loss, physical illness, and threat to his future health. He exists in a context. His family will have a role in his current predicament and in assisting his progress and he may require intervention from the GP and other community teams.

Dr Mike Cheshire, Consultant Physician in Medicine of the Elderly, Central Manchester and Manchester Children's Hospital Trust
The foundation of all good medicine is to get an accurate corroborated history. Check that this history is correct by reflecting what the patient, and carer if present, says and checking out detail. Be very clear about time relationships especially between the immobility, musculoskeletal pain, depression and retirement.

I am concerned about the phraseology of his complaints. Is this how he said it, or is it the clinician's interpretation and shorthand? Remember that first comments in an interview are very important and may carry up to 80% of the information that is needed to make a diagnosis. Note not only what a patient says but how they say it. Don't fall into the trap of paraphrasing and translating what they say into your notes. I see many patients in whose case notes the junior doctor will tell me that the patient says they are dysphasic, dysarthric, dyspnoeic. Of course they did not, that's the medical jargon for what the doctor thought the patient was describing. And it's often wrong! In that sense the problem that we are presented for analysis has all the rich language and description of the patient removed and is the doctor's thoughtful summary. If this summary or formulation is not correct then we will not solve the patient's problems. When presented with a complex problem explore the problem with the patient and then listen to the patient's narrative. That is where the answers will lie.

I am always wary of new presentations at retirement. So, although I accept that this may be the manifestation of loss of role, prestige, income, interest, this is also the time of life when severe and serious organic illness may present. As a physician I see my role as ensuring that his physical illness and disability is managed properly, actively and positively. Patients feel better psychologically when they are not ill physically.

The history given presents the diseases and problems as if it is an accurate summary. Of course that may be the case but as a secondary care specialist, I feel that it is my role to make sure (Box 4.1).

This patient is likely to have been referred to me by a GP colleague because of a concern that organic pathology is causing his symptoms, but that depression is suspected. I would make sure that I examine him very carefully, mentally and physically (Box 4.2).

In addition to preliminary investigations, which in this case have been done in primary care and the results sent to me, I would probably organize a chest X-ray, particularly if he has ever smoked. I would also X-ray his hips and back and assess whether the radiographs correlated with the level of pain and disability.

I then write down my assessment of his physical and mental state, paying attention to matching it with his history. It is very easy to produce the wrong solution for the wrong problem, and you want the correct solution for the correct problem. If you get this correct then management plans emerge with ease.

This is where things may get even more difficult. You may need to negotiate with the patient. What diagnosis or formulation will he accept? What do his wife and family feel?

Mr WH has a very negative outlook on life at present and in that setting only expects things to get worse. He was a high achiever and one formulation may be that he feels that life has finished.

If I think that the patient is depressed then I will ask the patient directly if they feel they are depressed and if so why. In my experience patients will usually admit and talk about depression if asked. They will also deny it

Box 4.1 Important areas to cover in the history

Is there anything to suggest that he has a systemic illness? Do not miss bone pain from Paget's disease, osteomalacia, hyperparathyroidism or metastases from carcinoma of the prostate.

Look for red flag symptoms: new pains especially disturbing sleep, anorexia, substantial weight loss, new symptoms such as a persistent cough, altered bowel habit.

Polymyalgia rheumatica with diurnal variations of stiffness and girdle pain is easy to miss if you do not ask about diurnal variation. How are you when you have been sitting? Is it difficult to sleep? And why is that? What is your worst time of the day and when are you at your best? I realize that the diurnal variation of depression is the same but careful listening may help distinguish between the two.

Has he lost weight? Does he suffer from sweats, shivers or rigors?

Is the pain in the hips and knees really in the hips and knees? Could it be referred from his back?

Even though he admits that he is hit-and-miss with his medication does he know how his diabetes control is?

I would enquire what medication is he prescribed and what he actually takes: they may be different and include over-the-counter and herbal preparations.

Does he smoke, does he drink alcohol, and if so how much?

Weepiness, thoughts of worthlessness, being unloved, hopelessness, life not worth living and of course suicidal intent or thoughts point to significant depression. Conversely patients who sleep and eat well are unlikely to be significantly depressed.

Does he still enjoys things, does he feel anxious, what are his ideas about the future? I would try to establish whether he had thoughts of harming himself. Did he have any other interests than work? What motivates and enthuses him?

I would ask what he thought was wrong with him.

sometimes and a more in-depth interview may be required talking about their thoughts, hopes and regrets, while watching carefully for alteration in eye contact or signs of tearfulness or alteration in the colour of their face. Careful pauses, giving permission to talk about uncomfortable issues, will help.

If I feel that the patient would benefit from an antidepressant then I will suggest this as a possibility, and then wait and see what he thinks. Sometimes a patient may reveal that he has been depressed before and understands the reasons why. If a patient denies the diagnosis it is always worth asking why.

Box 4.2 Examination

Does he look well? Does he look well cared for? How is his eye contact? What is the first thing that strikes you when you meet and talk with him?

Are there any features to suggest that he is physically ill? Is he pyrexial? What is his blood pressure (lying and standing)? Low blood pressure generally causes more symptoms than high blood pressure. Patients with postural hypotension will not walk because of light-headedness and a real fear of falling.

Does he have normal facial expression? Does he have any parkinsonian signs? Are the cranial nerves normal? Does he look depressed?

Does he have symmetrical or asymmetrical power, tone and sensation? And of course watch him walk. He is now spending time in a wheelchair: is that because he cannot walk or does not want to? Is that gait axatic, apraxic, unsteady, lop-sided? Fast, slow, upright, bent?

I would check his lymph node fields and his thyroid gland. Can you hear murmurs or abnormal chest signs? Is the abdomen normal or does he have a large liver or spleen?

How restricted and abnormal are his hips and knees?

If he looks depressed, I would very carefully assess his risk of self-harm.

Perhaps it's the apparent shame and cultural denial of depression. Of course they may not be depressed or may say something like 'I would not be depressed if I was well'; then ask what aspects of their illness would they like to be addressed.

One key question is how to manage his pain. It is most important to understand what his pain is due to and why it changed at retirement. Remember that pain causes depression and depression magnifies pain. If the pain is really osteoarthritis then although it may be difficult to move around, immobility will make the discomfort much worse, physiotherapy would be very important, perhaps even joint replacement. Careful attention to analgesia is crucial, but beware non-steroidal anti-inflammatory drugs (NSAIDs) in a patient with diabetes and potential renal impairment.

As for treatment and tablets for depression, I would suggest that they might be useful if that is what I thought but would not push the issue: 'Have a think and come back and see me again' often works. I would not be keen to refer on to a psychiatrist or other health professional without careful discussion with the GP. Patients with complex illness need to be managed in a team with a clear leader and in many cases that should be the GP. The GP may have information that I do not have access to which will substantially alter the management plans.

Finally, how is he to be managed in a physical, psychological and social context? First of all put them in order. Realize that relatively small issues may have a huge impact on the patient and that carefully formulating the whole picture may give insight into some relatively simple solutions. The interaction between health and social services, the family and the professional, the GP, the physician and psychiatrist are very important. In this case it is agreed that the GP will take the lead in co-ordinating care but it is not always clear. Because multiple agencies and people may be involved it can be a difficult exercise. It may be that as the problems are unravelled the primacy of the various agencies will alter; you will need to identify and adapt to this.

Case 4.3 Carers and families

Mr Le Lin P lives with his family above a Chinese takeaway which he set up 40 years ago when he first came to the UK. His two sons and their families now run the business and Mr LP feels he has nothing to contribute. His wife has severe osteoarthritis and has had hypertension for many years. She had a small stroke a year ago and Mr LP feels he has to watch her all the time. Members of her family have also noticed that she is getting increasingly forgetful recently and has, on occasions, wandered out of their flat. One of their teenage grandsons had to go and look for her. Mr LP has rarely consulted the GP but feels that he will have to go and see if something can be done for his wife, but he would also like to ask if he could have a tonic that would help him sleep and feel better with his lot, which he describes as 'an old sick couple'.

The GP is aware that Mr LP has rarely consulted in the past and seems to take no prescribed medication.

What issues would it be important to cover in the consultation and how might the couple be helped?

Dr Joanne Protheroe, General Practitioner and Clinical Research Fellow, Primary Care Research Group, School of Community Based Medicine, University of Manchester
My first impressions of this case are that there are a lot of issues to cover which cannot be achieved in a single consultation. We are talking about at least two patients here, both of whom have several needs that require assessment and management.

My first approach will be to take a detailed history and begin to develop a rapport with Mr LP. I am presuming that he is able to communicate directly in English, and not through an interpreter, although this may not be the case. It is not uncommon to have sensitive details communicated through a young granddaughter or other family member which, as Dr Waheed points out in Chapter 1, is not ideal.

Important details to uncover in the history include:

- Mr LP has rarely consulted before – what exactly has prompted him to come this time? Have other members of the family insisted? Has something particular happened?

- What does he expect to happen as a result of consulting? What are his concerns for his wife? What does he want to happen to her – is he concerned that he will not be able to continue to care for her at home – does he want to? How much help and support does he have from the family? Who is at home – which family members live together? What are his living conditions – he lives over a shop and his wife has severe osteoarthritis and has had a stroke – can she manage the stairs?

- I need to suggest that he attends next time with his wife next time in order to assess her physical and mental state. She should be being actively followed up by practice team since her stroke a year ago – but needs a further assessment for possible early dementia. This may result in a referral to a memory clinic or old-age psychiatrist.

- I need to assess his mood and mental state. He requests a 'tonic' to help him sleep. The use of 'tonics' is embedded in Chinese culture and we need to explore what he means by this. He is not on any prescribed medication – has he tried any herbal medication (use of substances such as St John's wort can have an effect on other prescribed medications)? The use of screening questions for depression may be helpful, such as 'During the last month have you been bothered by having little interest or pleasure in doing things?' Are his family circumstances (living above his shop, possibly crowded and no longer having a role to play in running the shop) contributing to his symptoms? If he is depressed it is important to consider his risk of self-harm and suicide.

- Given that Mr LP has rarely consulted previously, it would also be important to consider his physical health. Routine screening questions about his health, diet and lifestyle (weight, smoking, urine, alcohol, exercise) would be included and examinations (including blood pressure measurement) would be conducted as dictated by the history. Any blood tests that would be appropriate could be scheduled for a future appointment.

Management plans would be guided by the history, but possibilities could be discussed broadly with Mr LP at the first consultation. It is likely that social services could be involved to help with caring for his wife, if this is their wish. As mentioned, she may also require a referral to secondary care to a memory clinic or old-age psychiatrist depending on local provision. However, it must be stressed that Mrs P needs assessment first in order to discover the extent of her problems.

On first impressions it seems likely that Mr LP may be depressed. Depression is common in people who have caring responsibilities (Livingston *et al.* 1996). The severity of this depression should have been uncovered by the history and the use of an assessment schedule such as PHQ-9 (Kroenke *et al.* 2001; see also Chapter 7). It may be that he is suffering from mild depression exacerbated by his family and social circumstances. With plans to hopefully improve and manage his family and social problems, simple 'watchful waiting' as advocated by NICE Guidelines (NICE 2004) with further assessment within two weeks may be all that is required and this should be discussed with him.

Further treatments, if necessary, could be discussed at this or at follow-up consultations. Depending on the extent of his language abilities guided self-help or computerized cognitive behavioural therapy (CBT) (see Chapter 7) could be discussed, or he may prefer to be referred to the primary care mental health team for a brief psychological intervention over a period of 10–12 weeks.

If his depression is found to be of a moderate nature, or has not responded to the above management, the use of antidepressant medication should be discussed with Mr LP. Selective serotonin reuptake inhibitors (SSRIs) are appropriate medications in the treatment of moderate depression (possibly in addition to psychological therapy) but must be used in age-appropriate doses. Possible side effects should be discussed with Mr LP as should the likely length of treatment; in older patients antidepressants should be continued for at least four to six weeks before being considered ineffective.

Follow-up

A follow-up appointment should be arranged to see Mr LP with his wife with the intention of assessment of his wife's physical and mental problems (Alzheimer's Society 2007).

In addition a further follow-up of Mr LP alone to review his mood should be arranged within the next two weeks. Any investigations, including blood tests, suggested by the history should be organized.

The availability of all members of the primary health-care team for support and empathy for physical, psychological and social problems should be emphasized to Mr LP. He should be encouraged to contact the team again with any further concerns or problems.

Professor David Challis, Professor of Community Care Research, and Dr Jane Hughes, Lecturer in Community Care Research, Personal Social Services Research Unit, University of Manchester

Introduction

The approach taken by a social worker towards this client would be, as for any generic community-based professional, shaped by their level of specific training and experience of mental health services. The opportunities for response will be determined by the nature and flexibility of local services. Both are important variables in determining the response to the case described above. In this discussion, it is assumed that the social worker is experienced in old-age mental health services and has good working links with appropriate specialist services such as old-age psychiatry.

Assessment

In the assessment process, the social worker would take account of the overall family context – the needs of both Mrs Le Lin P (Mrs P) and Mr Le Lin P (Mr LP) who appears to have assumed the role of principal carer. The first step would be to establish that the couple would be eligible for social care support as deemed by the Fair Access to Care criteria (Department of Health 2002a). Next the social worker would determine the focus of assessment in the first instance. There are four immediate foci: Mrs P's physical health; her mental health; Mr LP's state of mind; and his role as principal carer of his wife. In respect of the latter he is entitled to a carer's assessment in his own right (Department of Health 2001a). Finally, there is the domain of the adequacy, appropriateness and sufficiency of the support services provided for both parties. In these circumstances it is likely that the initial assessment would focus on the needs of Mrs P. However, given the evidence of sleep disturbance and negative evaluation of his current situation, a concurrent assessment of Mr LP's mental state would be appropriate both in terms of his own health and sense of well-being as well as his capacity to continue as his wife's principal carer.

The introduction of the Single Assessment Process (SAP) (Department of Health 2002b) into localities in England has resulted in greater standardization and a requirement to address a range of specified domains of need in assessment. As part of this there should be a risk assessment which would encompass those factors which might jeopardize the possibility of Mrs LP remaining in her current familiar environment. Specifically these would appear to be:

- changing cognitive function in Mrs P
- poor-quality care for Mrs P
- fragility of the support for Mrs P which maintains her at home and risk of admission to a care home
- continued demands on Mr LP from the caring responsibility
- depression in Mr LP.

It would also be appropriate to offer to undertake a financial assessment to determine if the couple are receiving all the financial benefits to which they are entitled which could further enhance their support.

Treatment modalities

The risk assessment highlights how integral Mr LP's well-being is to his wife's care needs and therefore it is important to address both in the short term.

The goal of the resulting care package (Hughes *et al.* 2005) would be to achieve a new balance in the family arrangements, sustainable for the foreseeable future.

With regard to Mrs P, it will be important to consider a review of the support currently provided for her by her husband, both in terms of her personal care and structured daytime activities. A balance would need to be achieved between care provided in the family home and that provided outside at a facility such as a day centre to give her husband a break from his caring role. Moreover the capacity of the extended family to offer support to Mr and Mrs P should be taken into account. In establishing this care package it would be important to source an appropriate provider such as voluntary groups within the Chinese community in the locality. Where care managers have more flexible access to resources (Challis *et al.* 2002a) it might be possible to fund appropriate support from this local community. Elements of the care package provided by the social worker would accrue a charge levied by the local authority providing them and would be subject to regular review (Department of Health 2002a, 2002b).

The initial task with Mr LP is to address his symptoms which may be indicative of depression. Following an initial assessment, if appropriate, a treatment plan with both clinical and social components might be established. It is likely that this would focus the treatment and management of any long-term clinical condition and on his role as principal carer of his wife. In the longer term his needs might be most appropriately addressed by a formal assessment of his needs. The resulting care package might contain both practical components to support him in this role, such as providing him with time to pursue an interest outside the home by providing care for his wife, and a more therapeutic intervention designed to help him in reshaping and modifying his expectations of himself as a carer, possibly provided by the social worker. Engaging younger family members and also local voluntary organizations might also be considered in the care plan resulting from this carer's assessment.

Inter-agency working

From the perspective of the social worker, there are two aspects of this: linking with appropriate providers to provide care for Mrs P which respects her ethnic and cultural background and liaising with colleagues in the National Health Service regarding the health needs of both Mr and Mrs P. The latter requires links with both primary and secondary healthcare. Within primary care the principal contact would be the GP involving their contribution to the assessment of both Mr and Mrs P and particularly a review of their current medication. Screening for depression in Mr LP and dementia in Mrs P could appropriately be undertaken by the GP at this stage. Policy guidance suggests that this should be undertaken as part of the SAP, contributing to the assessment undertaken by the social worker in respect of Mrs P and initiating the process in respect of Mr LP (Department of Health 2002b).

A key issue would be the decision as to whether to refer either the husband and wife or both to specialist old-age psychiatry services. This could be made by either the GP or the social worker since many old-age psychiatry services accept referrals from a variety of sources (Challis *et al.* 2002b). For Mrs P such a referral could have a number of benefits, most notably a detailed assessment of her mental state and, if appropriate, medication recommendations to the GP and an assessment by an occupational therapist within the multidisciplinary team with regard to her ability to perform the instrumental activities of daily living. From this, appropriate guidance could be offered to her principal carer and paid carers who might be recruited to assist in this as part of the care package organized by the social worker. These interventions, together with the assessment undertaken by the social worker and the GP, could in sum constitute a comprehensive assessment within the SAP, designed to provide a detailed assessment of vulnerable older people with complex medical and social needs (Department of Health 2002b).

For Mr LP, the initial focus of the intervention of the specialist old-age psychiatry team, if Mr LP was so referred, would be the diagnosis and, if appropriate, treatment of depression. It is likely that a specialist clinician and a community psychiatric nurse would provide this in conjunction with the GP. In view of his role as principal carer to his wife and the risk factors identified in her care plan, regular contact would need to be maintained between the specialist service and the social worker organizing the care package to enable Mrs P to be cared for at home with continuity and cohesive support. A review meeting (Department of Health 2002a) involving the couple might be the appropriate mechanism to achieve this.

Links to national policy

There are several issues of national policy which are highlighted by this case. First, there is the configuration of services in the locality and what has been described as the 'Berlin Wall' dividing health and social care (Department of Health and Social Services 1998, para 6.5). The degree of integration between social care and old-age mental health services has been a concern to government and guidance has been issued (Department of Health 2001b). However, it must be noted that organizational integration between agencies does not necessarily lead to integration of services and response at the patient level (Reilly *et al.* 2003, Challis *et al.* 2006, Tucker *et al.* 2007). Related to this is the degree of multi-agency working in old-age psychiatry services, identified as essential in policy guidance (Department of Health 2001b) although the extent to which this has yet been achieved is variable (Philp and Appleby 2005, Tucker *et al.* 2007).

A second area of consideration is the eligibility of the family to receive social care support. Whilst this is shaped by the Fair Access to Care Services guidance (Department of Health 2002a), there remain local variations in the thresholds at which this is applied (CSCI 2007).

A third area where policy impacts upon this case is in respect of assessment. Historically, there was substantial variation in the components of a social care assessment for vulnerable older people (Stewart *et al.* 1999). The application of the SAP was designed to reduce duplication and increase standardization in assessment of older people (Department of Health 2002b). However, there remains much local variation in approach, particularly at the level of comprehensive assessment.

A fourth area of policy relevant to this case is the development of support for carers. Local authorities are required to provide carers with support and services to maintain their health. When there is reason to suspect risk to the sustainability of the caring role it is deemed to be good practice to offer a carer's assessment (Department of Health 2001a).

Finally, government has recently articulated the importance of services being able to respond more to the individual needs of people and has indicated the use of individual budgets as a mechanism (Department of Health 2006). In such a case as this, where mainstream services might be less appropriate for cultural reasons, this offers the potential to create a more flexible and bespoke care package for the couple in this case study.

Barriers and facilitating factors

This case study demonstrates that a number of factors influence the delivery of services for older people with mental health problems in a locality. These may be summarized as follows:

(1) The organization of old-age psychiatry services and in particular its com-position, links with social care services, community orientation and refer-ral policy.

(2) The location of the social worker will influence their ease of contact with colleagues in specialist old-age psychiatry services – they may be mem-bers of a multidisciplinary team or based in a local authority setting as members of a specialist older people's team or a generic adult services team.

(3) The training and experience of social workers in respect of mental health will vary both in terms of work experience and specialist knowledge.

(4) There are variations in the availability of local support services. With regard to social care there is evidence that where social workers had access to flexible resources care could be uniquely tailored to the circumstances of individual person (Challis *et al.* 1995, 2002).

Case 4.4 Ethnically sensitive management

Mr Afzal C worked as a bus driver until he had to retire due to ill-health in his late 50s. He has diabetes and low back pain. For 10 years he helped his eldest son in their shop and supported his younger children through college. A year ago, his son sold the business and moved further out of the city taking Mr AC and his wife to their new home. Mr AC is very isolated having lost his friends and feels guilty about wishing he was back in familiar surroundings. He believes his son is angry with him and he thinks that he expects him to be more grateful. He is having difficulty sleeping and feels anxious most of the time and guilty about being a burden.

Mr AC spent the past three months in Pakistan but on his return he felt just as miserable. He consulted a healer in Pakistan and was given some traditional remedies which didn't help, but he also saw a doctor who gave him tranquillizers just before his return to the UK. These certainly took the edge off how he felt.

How can the GP manage this man? Please discuss the cultural issues of relevance. How can Mr AC and his wife be supported?

Dr Greta Rait, General Practitioner and Senior Lecturer in Primary Care, Royal Free and University College Medical School, London

Context and assessment

Mr AC may present with his psychological symptoms, or they may be picked up during a review for his chronic disease (diabetes). Depression case finding in patients with diabetes is part of the English 2006 General Practitioner Quality and Outcomes Framework (BMA and NHS Employers 2006). As he moved to a new area one year ago, he may have registered with a new practice and be seeing a new GP. He may be seen on his own, or with his wife.

It is important to first listen to Mr AC's narrative and description of his life events, any expressed emotions and how he has responded. He clearly has had a number of significant events: loss of employment, chronic illnesses and loss of his social support and network. Having supported his family through their education and also at their work, he no longer views himself as useful, but rather as a burden on his family. It would be important to explore family dynamics and cultural expectations of family behaviour. Social isolation is a significant factor and an exploration of what he misses from his previous surroundings, for example community centres, shared language, place of worship, informal meeting with friends, is needed. It would be helpful to have Mr AC's wife's perspective on what is happening. Does she also have similar feelings, or is she coping well? As a GP I may know the family, but is important not to make assumptions. People from South Asian backgrounds can be assumed to have strong family support, but exploration of the family dynamic is important: this may or may not be not a supportive situation. There may be benefit in including the son in one of the consultations if Mr AC is happy with this, to get his perspective.

It is likely that English is Mr AC's second language and he may have good language skills. However, language used to describe psychological and emotional symptoms can be quite complex, and it can sometimes be helpful to have an interpreted consultation to allow for an exploration of these issues. It is also important that he grasps that understanding and treating psychological symptoms are part of the GP's role. Sometimes patients require permission to admit to psychological symptoms and open up to their doctors.

It is useful to explore whether religion plays a significant role in Mr AC's life and whether this can be included in the discussion of how best to address his feelings and manage his isolation and loneliness.

He has used some medications: traditional remedies that did not work and some tranquillizers that did. It is important to find out what medication he is still taking. It is easy to make assumptions, e.g. older people who are Muslim do not drink. Again prefacing questions about alcohol with an introduction about why you are asking and that they are questions that everyone is asked helps make questions on sensitive topics acceptable.

Psychological disorders and chronic disease are often associated and it is important to understand his feelings about his diabetes and back pain. Did the depression occur before or after the diagnoses? Does he have particular health concerns?

As with all patients it is helpful to use a standard tool to assess depression such as the Geriatric Depression Scale (GDS) which performs reasonably with people from South Asian backgrounds (Rait *et al.* 2000). Risk assessment is important. Some people with strong religious faith find questions about suicide difficult and it is useful to preface these with a short introduction to why the questions are being asked.

Treatments

There are a number of key areas that the GP needs to assess. First there is the severity of any depression and/or anxiety, and use of rating scales such as the GDS will help with assessing the severity of Mr AC's depression and/or anxiety.

Second, Mr AC's interpretation of his symptoms, his health beliefs and what input he wants must be ascertained. He may acknowledge that he is 'miserable' or the GP may have to help him reattribute his other symptoms, for example of poor sleep. It is always helpful to give people written information about their illness, in the language that they prefer. The discussion of the diagnosis needs to be handled sensitively and issues around stigma addressed. This may need to be revisited over follow-up consultations. The treatment options may be discussed at this initial consultation or over a series of consultations. Mr C may not want any input other than seeing his GP, and it may take time to review and accept other treatment, if indicated.

Mr AC may want some informal support and this may be via a religious leader or through a community centre. These may help with the social isolation. However we need to be aware that sometimes people do not want to share their symptoms with other members of the community, as they are concerned about confidentiality. Age Concern has initiatives for people from black and ethnic minority backgrounds. MIND, a mental health charity (see also Chapter 7) has a good overview of diversity issues, and a list of useful organizations across the UK. Local councils will usually have lists of information about community groups (e.g. luncheon clubs, leisure and cultural activities). He may benefit from local activities and there may be volunteering schemes he could join, or voluntary organizations that could help with activities. Ahmed Lambat discusses one such approach in the following commentary.

Depression may benefit from some form of psychological therapy. This needs to be explained clearly. In some localities there are culturally sensitive counselling services. Some practices will have practice-based counselling, which would be local and convenient. The therapy may extend to his family if needed. Computerized cognitive behavioural therapy (CBT) could be beneficial if his language skills were good and if this was acceptable to him.

Depending on severity, response to psychological therapy or patient preference the GP may consider pharmacological intervention. As the patient is probably on medication for diabetes and back pain, it is important to review current medications, avoid polypharmacy and consider interactions.

His physical condition (diabetes and back pain) needs to be optimized. He may benefit from peer support or from participating in a self-management programme (see Expert Patients' Programme 2007) to improve his confidence in managing his own conditions, and this may help reduce his anxiety symptoms. He needs regular review of his diabetes, which may be through a practice-based diabetes clinic. Exercise would benefit his physical and psychological health; he could be referred for exercise on prescription if available, or keep-fit classes for older people.

It is important to ensure regular review and continuity of care. Primary care allows for the development of long-term relationships, monitoring of treatment and review of symptoms. This may be carried out by the GP or the practice nurse.

If Mr AC's mood fails to improve or worsens then it would be necessary to discuss his care with the local old-age psychiatry team or community mental health team. In some cases they would only provide advice but they might also need to review him and discuss a shared care plan. Liaison is important and clear explanations are needed for patients regarding the roles of different professionals and treatment options.

Ahmed I. Lambat, Manager and Social Work Practice Teacher, Manchester
Fernando (1995) writes: 'the voluntary sector has an important, perhaps crucial, role to play in the provision of mental health services in a multi-ethnic society'.

Longsight/Moss Side Community Project in Manchester, UK, is a voluntary sector organization with over a decade's experience of working with and on behalf of older South Asian persons, their carers and South Asian women with mental health needs. I will describe our approach to supporting South Asian persons, our attempts to work with health and social care professionals and the challenges that remain.

Like many small voluntary organizations, and despite poor funding, we adopt a 'slow social work' (Killic 2004) approach to supporting our service users. In the case of Mr AC, our outreach worker would visit the family a number of times to get to know them and to allow them to learn about her role as an outreach worker and to decide on how best she can support them. She would encourage the family to discuss Mr AC's feeling of isolation, his perceptions of his son's feelings towards him, his physical and emotional health as well as their other needs including social care, welfare benefits and housing. Although Mr AC accessed help in Pakistan, he may be reluctant to do so in the UK for fear of stigma, and for fear of further 'annoying' his son. The quality time spent by the outreach worker with the service-user and his family often serves to clarify misunderstanding, improves communication and helps the service-user become better informed about health and social care services available and how these could help improve their quality of life. This then helps the service-user to accept that outside help is necessary.

The outreach worker offers to be present at the GP consultation to ensure that the feelings are discussed and acknowledged by both parties, that there is a discussion of medication, and that alternative treatment approaches such as talking therapy are considered. Equally, the outreach worker would look to the GP for support in encouraging the service-user/patient to consider other support. The outreach worker would also seek to share with the GP and other relevant professionals her knowledge and understanding of cultural and religious issues as well as alternative sources of support available to Mr AC such as social support from community organizations, places of worship and luncheon clubs and about culturally/religiously appropriate mental health services.

'Faith and religious groups can offer a powerful opportunity to build positive social networks for people with mental health problems, and they can be particularly important for some ethnic minority groups.' (Social Exclusion Unit 2004.) The outreach worker with her in-depth knowledge of the South Asian communities would assist Mr AC to identify and access support from appropriate faith and religious groups. The outreach worker would also inform Mr AC and his family about other support which would help him reduce his social isolation, for example by joining a luncheon club. If necessary, support would be provided with travel arrangements (bus pass/travel vouchers). If day care was considered to be more appropriate then the outreach worker would make a referral to the social services department for a community care assessment. A carer's assessment would be made for Mrs C.

Mrs C and her son would be encouraged to join a carers' support group where they would be able to meet with other carers and learn about services available to support them.

Supporting professionals and commissioners of mental health services

Our organization attempts to inform the work of social and health-care professionals (including mental health) with South Asians in the following ways.

- Accompanying service-users/patients on appointments and review meetings to share our knowledge and understanding of peoples' needs.
- Organizing events. Examples locally have included a Faith and Mental Health conference in Manchester and an Older South Asians and Mental Health event as part of the World Mental Health Day.
- Working in partnership, for example, a pilot programme for older South Asian women with mental health needs along with the local Mental Health Trust.
- Contributing to strategy: contributing to development of policies to help improve the availability and uptake of culturally and religiously appropriate mental health services.

Challenges

Since the introduction of the National Service Framework for Mental Health in 1999, much has been produced by way of research reports, guidelines, policies and strategies nationally and locally (see for example Department of Health 2005). Yet, as the Minister for State for Health Services recently commented in a letter to senior health service managers, 'the quality of mental health care for BME (black and minority ethnic) communities in England is not acceptable'.

A number of challenges still remain for a voluntary sector organization such as ours and include:

- poor understanding of depression and other mental health conditions and of health and social care services amongst South Asians

- stigma, language barriers and the attitude ('we know best', colour-blind approach) of some health and social care professionals preventing service-users from seeking services
- poor understanding of cultural and religious needs by health and social care professionals
- unwillingness of some health and social care professionals to work with colleagues from the voluntary sector
- lack of funding resulting in, for example, limited provision of talking therapies, negligible provision such as mental health drop-ins for South Asian men
- busy health and social care professionals not being able to spend in-depth time with older persons and their families
- the confusion between primary and secondary care and the role of the various professionals
- over-prescription of antidepressants, especially for South Asian women.

Our organization continues to raise these issues with commissioners of mental health care.

Editors' comments

We feel that these cases highlight the following points.

Notes on Case 4.1

- Assessment of patients who appear to have a 'dual diagnosis' requires an in-depth assessment of both problems.
- Defining the type of elderly drinker (for example symptomatic versus dependent drinking) can shape management strategies and predict outcome.
- Treatment of both depression and alcohol misuse should be offered, with referral to specialist alcohol workers if available and if acceptable to the patient.
- With potentially several agencies involved, managing the physical damage from drinking alcohol should not be overlooked.

Notes on Case 4.2

- Presentation of physical symptoms may be due to somatization of distress; alternatively, physical symptoms of organic pathology may be exacerbated by coexistent depression. A full history and examination is needed to separate the two.
- It is important to check for red flag symptoms (for example anorexia, altered bowel habit) even if the patient is clearly depressed.

- It is important to acknowledge a person's distress, whatever its underlying cause.
- Antidepressants can be helpful in pain management, especially when linked to depression.
- The GP and physician may have overlapping roles and collaboration is vital to avoid duplication of care or conflicting advice.

Notes on Case 4.3

- Racial and ethnic background can affect the presentation of depression and acceptability of depression as a diagnosis.
- Several rating scales have translations into languages other than English.
- Depression is common in carers of people with chronic physical disease or mental health problems such as dementia. It is a hidden, overlooked problem. In England care-givers have a right to an assessment of their own needs
- The Single Assessment Process (SAP) offers a broad standardized assessment including risk and is intended to avoid duplicated information.
- The care package needs to address the whole family's needs and to achieve a new balance in family arrangements, and must be sustainable.

Notes on Case 4.4

- Although people from South Asian backgrounds often have strong family support, one cannot assume this is the case.
- Involving family members as interpreters has both advantages and drawbacks.
- The role played by traditional remedies in this family must be explored, together with attitudes to Western medicine.
- A knowledge of local voluntary sector agencies specific to particular cultural or ethnic groups is vital.
- Referral to a local group may be more effective and appropriate than prescription of antidepressants.
- Provided they can be understood, standard psychological interventions can be applied to different ethnic groups.

REFERENCES

Alzheimer's Society (2007) *Working_with_People_with_Dementia*. Available online at www.alzheimers.org.uk/

Beck A. T., Wright F. D., Newman C. F., Liese B. S. (1993) *Cognitive Theory of Substance Abuse*. New York: Guilford Press.

Blow F. C. (2000) Treatment of older women with alcohol problems: meeting the challenge for a special population. *Alcohol Clin. Exp. Res.* **24**, 1257–66.

BMA and NHS Employers. (2006) *Revisions to the GMS Contract, 2006/7: Delivering Investment in General Practice*. London: British Medical Association.

Bower P., Gilbody S. (2005) Stepped care in psychological therapies: access, effectiveness and efficiency – narrative literature review. *Br. J. Psychiatry* **186**, 11–17.

Challis D., Darton R., Johnson L., Stone M., Traske K. (1995) *Care Management and Health Care of Older People: The Darlington Community Care Project*. Aldershot, UK: Arena Press.

Challis D., Chesterman J., Luckett R., Stewart K., Chessum R. (2002a) *Care Management in Social and Primary Health Care*. Aldershot, UK: Ashgate.

Challis D., Reilly S., Hughes J., *et al.* (2002b) Policy, organization and practice of specialist old age psychiatry in England. *Int. J. Geriatr. Psychiatry* **17**, 1018–26.

Challis D., Stewart K., Donnelly M., Weiner K., Hughes J. (2006) Care management for older people: does integration make a difference? *J. Interprof. Care* **20**, 335–48.

CSCI (2007) *The State of Social Care in England*. London: Commission for Social Care Inspection.

Department of Health (2001a) *Carers and Disabled Children Act 2000: A Practitioner's Guide to Carers' Assessment*. London: HMSO.

Department of Health (2001b) *National Service Framework for Older People*. London: HMSO.

Department of Health (2002a) *Fair Access to Care Services: Guidance on Eligibility Criteria for Adult Social Care*, LAC (2002)13. London: HMSO.

Department of Health (2002b) *Guidance on the Single Assessment Process for Older People*, HSC2002/001: LAC (2002)1, London: HMSO.

Department of Health (2005) *Delivering Race Equality in Mental Health Care: An Action Plan for Reform Inside and Outside Services*. London: The Stationery Office.

Department of Health (2006) *Our Health, Our Care, Our Say: A New Direction for Community Services*. London: The Stationery Office.

Department of Health and Social Services (1998) *Modernizing Social Services*. London: HMSO.

Devanand D. P. (2002) Comorbid psychiatric disorders in late life depression. *Biol. Psychiatry* **52**, 236–42.

Drummond C., Oyefoso A., Phillips T., *et al.*: Alcohol Needs Assessment Research Project (ANARP) (2004) *The 2004 National Alcohol Needs Assessment for England*. London: Department of Health.

Expert Patients' Programme (2007) *Home Page*. Available online at www.expert patients.nhs.uk

Fernando S. (1995) *Mental Health in a Multi-Ethnic Society: A Multidisciplinary Handbook*. London: Routledge.

Hughes J., Sutcliffe C., Challis D. (2005) Social work. In *Standards in Dementia Care*, ed. A. Burns. Abingdon, UK: Taylor and Francis, pp. 00–00.

Institute of Alcohol Studies (1999) *Alcohol and the Elderly*. St Ives, UK: Institute of Alcohol Studies.

Killic C. (2004) Slowly but surely. *Community Care* 11–17 November 2004. Available online at www.communitycare.co.uk.

Kroenke K., Spitzer R. L., Williams J. B. (2001) The PHQ-9: validity of a brief depression severity measure. *J. Gen. Intern. Med.* **16**, 606–13.

Moyer A., Finney J. W., Swearingen C. E., Vergun P. (2002) Brief interventions for alcohol problems: a meta-analytic review of controlled investigations in treatment-seeking and non-treatment-seeking populations. *Addiction* **97**, 279–92.

NICE (2004). *Depression: Management of Depression in Primary and Secondary Care,* Clinical Guideline No.23. London: National Institute for Health and Clinical Excellence.

Pettinati H. M. (2004) Antidepressant treatment of co-occurring depression and alcohol dependence. *Biol. Psychiatry* **56**, 785–92.

Philp I., Appleby L. (2005) *Securing Better Mental Health Services for Older Adults.* London: Department of Health.

Rait G., Burns A., Baldwin R., *et al.* (2000) Validating screening instruments for cognitive impairment in older South Asians in the United Kingdom. *Int. J. Geriatr. Psychiatry* **15**, 54–62.

Reilly S., Challis D., Burns A., Hughes J. (2003) Does integration really make a difference? A comparison of old age psychiatry services in England and Northern Ireland. *Int. J. Geriatr. Psychiatry* **18**, 887–93.

Sacks S. (2000) Co-occurring mental and substance use disorders: promising approaches and research issues. *Substance Use and Misuse* **35**, 2061–93.

Scogin F., McElreath L. (1994) Efficacy of psychosocial treatments for geriatric depression: a quantitative review. *J. Counsel. Clin. Psychol.* **62**, 69–74.

Social Exclusion Unit, (2004) *Action on Mental Health: A Guide to Promoting Social Inclusion.* London: Office of the Deputy Prime Minister.

Sullivan L. E., Fiellin D. A., O'Connor P. G. (2005) The prevalence and impact of alcohol problems in major depression: a systematic review. *Am. J. Med.* **118**, 330–41.

Stewart K., Challis D., Carpenter I., Dickinson E. (1999) Assessment approaches for older people receiving social care: content and coverage. *Int. J. Geriatr. Psychiatry* **14**, 147–56.

Tucker S., Baldwin R., Hughes J., *et al.* (2007) Old age services mental health services in England: implementing the National Service Framework for Older People. *Int. J. Geriatr. Psychiatry* **22**, 211–17.

5

Management of late-life depression across primary and secondary care: case studies UK

In the next three case commentaries we asked our contributors to comment on more complicated cases where input from both primary and secondary health care and social care would be necessary.

Case 5.1 Depression with psychotic features

Mrs Paulette B is an African-Caribbean lady who came over to the UK 50 years ago with her husband. She raised six children who have all done very well and all except one live in different parts of the UK. When her husband died, Mrs PB threw herself into her work with the local church, helping run a group for young women and teaching in the Sunday School. For the last three months she has been off her food, unable to concentrate, less interested in things and reluctant to go to church, fearing that she will bring some calamity onto the congregation.

In the last two weeks, she has been aware of a man's voice warning her to stay at home and to avoid answering the telephone as her thoughts will be recorded. Initially she thought this might be her husband's voice but has now become convinced that it is the voice of the vicar and so when he called on her last week, she spoke to him through the door. She told him she knew that she had committed 'the unforgivable sin'. She also told him about the voice and how it is getting more upsetting and telling her that she is being watched and that God will punish her and the whole congregation.

What could her increasingly bizarre thoughts represent? What action should be taken, and why?

How would the GP and psychiatrist work together with this patient?

Professor Helen Lester, General Practitioner and Professor of Primary Care, School of Community Based Medicine, University of Manchester

Depression is relatively common in people over 65 and most GPs will be treating approximately 30 patients with depression at any given time. Seeing an

Integrated Management of Depression in the Elderly, ed. C. Chew-Graham, R. Baldwin and A. Burns. Published by Cambridge University Press. © Cambridge University Press 2008.

elderly person with psychotic depression, is, however, is a relatively rare occurrence in primary care, though one that needs to be taken seriously and managed promptly because of the distress and significant risk of suicide.

An important general principal for the primary care clinician is to listen to the family. This applies to conditions and circumstances beyond mental health issues, but is perhaps most pertinent in this area of care. It is likely that one of Mrs PB's children, perhaps alerted by the pastor, contacted the GP to express their worries about their mother. In these circumstances, although patient confidentiality is always extremely important, the GP would listen to the close family and discuss relevant issues, and arrange to make an urgent home visit when, hopefully, a family member could be present to open the door as well as expand on the history. Ideally, a family member would also have had an opportunity to explain to their mother that the GP would be calling round, since a sudden and unexpected arrival might aggravate the situation and mean Mrs PB was less likely to want to discuss her problems.

The GP would initially spend some time reassuring Mrs PB that they were there to help. Continuity of care is one of the key strengths of primary care and hopefully the GP would be able use this, building on their previous relationship and knowledge of each other, to gain Mrs PB's trust and confidence.

The GP would then want to take a detailed history, focussing particularly on affective symptoms of depression and the psychotic features such as the disordered thoughts and auditory hallucinations. Although there are few likely differential diagnoses, the GP would need to ask about physical health issues, consider whether Mrs PB was in fact experiencing the early stages of dementia and specifically check what medication was being prescribed and bought over the counter, and explore current alcohol consumption. The GP would also want to make a note of how well Mrs PB was looking after herself, assessed through changes in weight and her personal appearance, which is also likely to be mirrored by the state of cleanliness of the house. Once again, comparison with her appearance during previous consultations and possibly previous home visits would be helpful when assessing her current mental and physical state.

It is unclear how recently Mrs PB's husband died, but the mood-congruent hallucination is far more suggestive of psychotic depression than a pathological grief reaction. It is, however, also important to be sensitive to Paulette's African-Caribbean culture in this context and to clarify with family members if any of her thoughts, feelings or actions might be considered appropriate in the culture in which she was raised.

Above all, however, the GP would want to assess whether Mrs PB had any ideas of self-harm, and, if she had, whether she had taken any steps towards making these real, such as storing up tablets or writing letters to her children. They would also want to explore the difficult but critical issue of whether she had any notions about harming others, perhaps the pastor or the congregation.

The GP should gain the views of family members on how they felt their mother had been, and request their support, if required, in persuading their mother to accept help. Ideally, Mrs PB would recognize that the distressing thoughts and voices represented an illness, but it is possible that she might be resistant to the idea that she was unwell and needed treatment.

After a consultation that could have taken up to an hour, the GP would need to decide on the degree of urgency in requesting an opinion from secondary mental health services. Different geographical areas have different 'first contact/crisis' teams, but ideally, the GP would want to organize an assessment by an experienced mental health practitioner within no more than two days and on the same day if there were any significant safety concerns. Ideally, the GP would also arrange to be present at that visit, in terms of information sharing, reassurance for Mrs PB and formulating a joint management plan, although the demands of primary care mean that this would not always be possible and communication between primary care and secondary care specialist might have to be by telephone.

If Mrs PB was admitted to hospital, primarily because of concerns for her own and/or others' safety, or because it was felt she would benefit from electroconvulsive treatment (ECT), the GP's role would become one of supporting the family and liaising with secondary care about discharge and follow-up arrangements, especially after inpatient admission. She would need time to regain trust in her body and mind and reconnect with her friends and neighbours, many of whom might hold negative views about people who have had a mental illness. After discharge, the GP could help through ensuring clarity around treatment strategies and follow-up, keeping secondary care informed of any subsequent developments and by offering a listening ear and unconditional advocacy in the middle of a confusing and distressing life event.

If, however, the decision was made to support Mrs PB at home, and to start, for example, antidepressant monotherapy, the GP would need to reassess her mental and physical state regularly through weekly home visits and, in conjunction with secondary care, assess side effects and the effectiveness of her treatment. Some primary care teams might also have access to a primary care graduate mental health worker, who could help liaison with the voluntary sector if additional social support was required and, as Mrs PB's mental state improved, the GP might be able to involve an experienced practice nurse in terms of follow-up and assessment of mood and medication. The GP would become, in effect, the 'station master' keeping all the agencies involved communicating in an effective and timely manner, with Mrs PB's needs at the centre. Finally, the GP would continue to have an important role during the recovery phase by helping Mrs PB to understand the importance of continuing her medication once she felt like her old self.

Dr Harry Allen, Consultant in Old-Age Psychiatry, Manchester Mental Health and Social Care Trust

Assessment

The presenting features that Mrs PB has are immediately obviously serious. The symptoms she has may be command hallucinations, and although the instructions are benign at the moment, they may not always remain so. This might be a red flag symptom. How did she come to the attention of the GP? Was it the pastor who raised concerns, or perhaps another member of the congregation? Such patients occasionally present to the GP even though they may not think of themselves as ill. In this situation, the person alerting the health services may prove to be an invaluable ally in trying to gain access to Mrs PB so as to perform a preliminary assessment.

The assessment, which may have to be facilitated by the informant, needs to be urgently completed. It is unlikely that Mrs PB can be coaxed to the surgery, and a home visit by the GP will probably be required. Before visiting, it would be advisable to try to gather some additional information. Does she have a previous psychiatric diagnosis? Is there any history of aggression to others? Is the area safe to visit at this time of day? Does the visitor have any training in self-defence or breakaway techniques?

If the GP visits the patient the history of the symptoms, their onset and development should be elicited. What risk does Mrs PB pose to herself at this time? Has she developed ideas that would encourage her to end her life given that she considered herself to be such a risk to her congregation? Are her auditory hallucinations giving her instructions, and if so, what are the instructions? Can the pastor persuade her not to act on the instructions? Is she considering harming others? Has she accumulated a stock of tablets over the last few months with which to end her life? If these symptoms are present, and considered to indicate immediate risk to her life, the GP might consider a call to the duty approved social worker with a view to a Mental Health Act assessment immediately. If getting a second medical opinion would involve an unacceptable delay, then Section 4 of the Mental Health Act could be used (see Chapter 7 for links to the Mental Health Act 1983).

The GP should also consider the possibility of physical illness. Has there been a change in her physical health? Once the GP has considered these risk factors, then appropriate action can be taken. Such an assessment is required so as to be able to determine the correct step in the NICE stepped care model (NICE 2004a). In emergency situations, this could include requesting a domiciliary consultation with a view to detention in hospital. If the clinical features do not indicate such an emergency, then an urgent referral to the local community mental health service should be the next step. This clinical scenario would require a step 4 response (see Chapter 2), involving mental health specialists including crisis response teams. This service should be able to act on the referral rapidly, through a triage system, which can identify such urgent cases, and respond in a timely manner.

Whatever the method, it is likely that the system will identify this scenario as being urgent, and that an assessment by specialist in old-age psychiatry is required. The specialist will need to visit and gain entry to the house, possibly with the help of a trusted friend or relative or perhaps the GP, and conduct an interview. Questions should cover the psychological aspects of Mrs PB's condition, including her mood, feelings of hopelessness, or helplessness and guilt. She should be encouraged to talk about the threat she feels she poses to her congregation and what she may be planning to do about it. She should be coaxed to talk about any suicidal ideas, and the preparation for any attempt she may have made. Has she accumulated a stockpile of tablets as an insurance policy for when she needs to end her life? What keeps her going, or prevents her from acting on her plans just yet? The specialist should find out about the biological features of her sleep, appetite and weight, her energy, and the way her mood varies as the day passes. The social effects of her condition should be explored, with questions about her withdrawal, reduction in functioning and activity, and loss of contact with her friends and the church. Is she getting basic necessities into the house? Does anyone have regular access to her? Finally, she should be asked about her hallucinations, though the timing of these questions needs to be judged carefully so as to avoid raising them too early before trust has been gained and too late when she has become tired or irritable. What form do the voices take? Are they giving her instructions? Are they ignorable? Are they talking directly to her?

Once the specialist has completed the assessment, s/he and the GP should agree on a diagnosis and management plan. Ideally the specialist would meet the GP back at the surgery where the specialist is a regular visitor (if a liaison model of primary–secondary care operates), and a plan can be constructed. The symptoms described here may indicate depressive disorder with mood congruent psychotic features, or possibly a late-onset schizophreniform psychosis. The treatment plan should include further investigations including physical examination and blood sampling. Mrs PB may not agree to have blood tests done at the initial presentation, but every effort should be made to persuade her to have a physical examination. Blood tests may have to be deferred until a later date if the patient will not agree, but we should avoid an unnecessary delay in treatment and they must not be overlooked later on.

Mrs PB will require the help and support of her friends and family in agreeing to and maintaining treatment. Gaining their trust and involvement is essential, whilst working within the bounds of confidentiality and as far as Mrs PB will allow. She will have to be persuaded that her condition requires medical help. The involvement of a member of the community mental health team such as a community psychiatric nurse will assist here. Concordance with medication is essential if she is to have the best chance of recovery.

If the preferred diagnosis is of depressive disorder with mood congruent psychotic features, then treatment should include both an antidepressant, and an antipsychotic. The choice of antidepressant should depend on the type of symptoms Mrs PB shows. If she has predominantly withdrawn apathetic symptoms, then an antidepressant with noradrenergic reuptake inhibition may help. If she is tense and irritable, then serotonergic reuptake inhibition should be the primary mode of action. The team involved should consider how the medication is going to be provided for Mrs PB. Who will supervise, and what quantities will be available at any time for her? Prescriptions can be left with the chemist, and even daily doses can be dispensed if necessary. Blister packs, or a similar packaging, can help the community psychiatric nurse monitor concordance with the medication regime. Nonetheless some patients will sometimes dispose of their medication however it is provided, and mislead those involved.

The choice of antipsychotic has been made more complex recently consequent upon the Medicines and Healthcare Products Regulatory Agency's advice (MHRA 2005). This advice is that where patients have cerebrovascular risks factors, atypical antipsychotics should be used with caution. The risks must be weighed against the need for a tolerated antipsychotic that does not induce the metabolic syndrome.

Psychotic depression can be treatment resistant, and the situation must be kept under regular review. If progress is not being made after four weeks, and doses are at maximum tolerated level, then early consideration of ECT may be required. This will almost certainly involve admission to hospital. ECT treatment can be successful in psychotic depression. The difficulty will become one of maintaining remission. Some patients can gain significant benefit from psychologist involvement during the recovery phase. Insight into the condition can be encouraged and this can help with concordance.

Management of this patient requires a collaborative approach between primary and secondary care, and close communication between Mrs PB and relatives involved in supporting her at home.

Case 5.2 Risk of self-harm

Mrs Gladys H had cared for her husband with Parkinson's disease for the past five years. They had been married 49 years and their only son had been killed in car crash 28 years ago. This had led to Mrs GH having what she referred to as a 'breakdown'. She was otherwise well, apart from osteoarthritis of the knees and low back pain, for which she took occasional NSAIDs. For the past six months Mr H had been confined to a bed or chair and latterly she had found it difficult to lift him. He had fallen twice and she had needed to call an ambulance. She wasn't sleeping and felt exhausted all day, often just sitting crying. Despite the help of carers twice a day, she had agreed with her social worker that she should try him out in a nursing home and he had been admitted three days ago for a trial period. Without him she felt bereft, guilty that she could no longer cope with him, and she told the practice nurse that she felt she couldn't go on. She referred to an article she had read in the newspaper about 'mercy killing' and how some countries allow it, but the nurse is not clear whether she is referring to herself or her husband.

How should the risk of self-harm be assessed? Please discuss the responsibilities of the GP, social worker and psychiatrist in the management of this lady. What are the barriers and facilitators to them all working together?

Dr Simon Cocksedge, General Practitioner and Lecturer in General Practice, University of Manchester
Mrs GH requires *assessment* today and then *management* over the next few weeks. Assessment of risk and needs should probably be by her GP, though a community psychiatric nurse might fulfil this role, depending on local team-working arrangements. Management will be need to be shared between primary care, social services and psychiatric services.

Assessment

Initial assessment needs to confirm, first, if Mrs GH has depression and, if so, how severe it is, and second, if she is actively suicidal. Mrs GH has several factors in her history suggestive of severe depression which need exploring:

- Precipitating event – husband's admission to nursing home
- Pressure from current life events – husband's ongoing illness/deterioration
- Past history – 'breakdown' following bereavement
- Coexisting medical condition – chronic osteoarthritis
- Current symptoms affecting her life – sleep disturbance, fatigue, sense of guilt, thoughts of death, psychomotor retardation.

Further questioning must establish if she is suicidal and may reveal other symptoms (such as low self-esteem, feelings of hopelessness, poor concentration, confirmation of depressed mood, reduced interest). Her feelings concerning suicide must be explored directly – there is no evidence that asking about suicide makes self-harm more likely. For Mrs GH, this might include exploration of what she meant in telling the practice nurse first that 'she felt she couldn't go on' and second about 'mercy killing'. Mrs GH has risk factors for suicide (see Box 5.1) – old age, social isolation and depression.

It is crucial to distinguish between suicidal ideation ('I've thought about suicide') and suicidal intent ('I'm planning suicide'). Useful questions (see

---

Box 5.1 Risk factors for suicide

- Male > female
- Age >40 years
- Living alone/social isolation
- Divorced > widowed > never married > married
- Unemployment
- Chronic or serious physical illness
- Past psychiatric history
- Recent admission to psychiatric hospital
- History of suicide attempt/self-harm
- Alcohol/drug abuse
- Certain professions – vets, pharmacists, farmers, doctors
- Depression
- Personality disorder

Source: Chantal *et al.* (2005).

Box 5.2 Useful questions about suicidal ideas and plans

- Do you feel you have a future?
- Do you feel that life's not worth living?
- Do you ever feel completely hopeless?
- Do you ever feel you'd be better off dead and away from it all?
- Have you ever made any plans for suicide (if drug overdose – have you handled the tablets)?
- Have you ever made an attempt to take your own life?
- What prevents you from doing it?
- Have you made any arrangements for your affairs after your death?

Source: Chantal *et al.* (2005).

Box 5.2) are 'What stops you?' (for ideation), and 'Exactly how and when are you going to end it all?' (for intent).

The severity of Mrs GH's depression can be quantified using a questionnaire (such as the PHQ-9, as described in Chapter 7), taking into account her cultural background which might affect, for example, her degree of somatization or language used to describe mood. Examination should include general appearance (especially self-neglect, weight loss, evidence/smell of alcohol), assessment of mood, exclusion of psychotic symptoms, physical examination, and blood tests for a physical cause of her tiredness/low mood.

Management

Management of Mrs GH depends on the outcome of assessment. If she is *actively suicidal*, with clear intent, then she is at significant risk (step 4 of the stepped care model: see Chapter 2) – immediate intervention by specialist mental health services is required. She should not be left alone and assessment should be requested urgently by either a psychiatrist or a mental health crisis resolution team, depending on local availability. This may result in admission to hospital (perhaps enforced by Mental Health Act section if necessary), or intensive support in the community (perhaps with several daily contacts by community mental health team (CMHT) members).

If Mrs GH has *moderate or severe depression* and is *not at immediate risk of suicide* (ideation, not intent; step 3 of the stepped care model) then she should be managed in primary care in liaison with mental health and social services. In this situation, *medical management* of Mrs GH is based on antidepressant medication for a minimum of six months after remission, prescribed in small quantities initially (7–14 days), with full explanation, and monitoring of concordance. GP review will be needed at least every two weeks at first, then two to four weekly for three months.

Social care is initially about acute phase support, which might involve daily contact in person or by telephone, in liaison with any family members. Assessment and management would focus on both Mrs GH and her husband who both need to come to terms with his illness and its implications. For Mr H, a review of care with a multidisciplinary approach, perhaps involving a rehabilitation programme (including occupational therapy and physiotherapy), might lead to an assessment period (about four weeks) back at home incorporating day care, respite and intensive social support. This might ease the transition from living at home to residential care for both Mr and Mrs H. For Mrs GH, a carer's assessment is needed, again involving a multidisciplinary approach in which engaging her constructively despite her depression will be essential. In the short term, she may be helped by going to the nursing home daily, having a meal there, and perhaps sharing in activities or outings.

Psychological treatment for Mrs GH will be helpful to explore and address her feelings of guilt/bereavement. Initially, this might be undertaken by a suitably trained social worker, the CMHT, or a practice counsellor (PC). Medium-term psychological management, such as cognitive behavioural therapy or counselling, might be offered via CMHT or PC.

All care for Mrs GH, medical, social or psychological, will be time-limited and will require reassessment, again with multidisciplinary liaison between GP, social worker, CMHT and PC. If Mrs GH's depression becomes more severe, or is unresponsive to social care and medical treatment in primary care, assessment by a psychiatrist will be needed. Barriers to effective management of Mrs GH and her husband include the availability of social, medical and psychological services locally, along with funding for intensive home support if needed. Close liaison between service providers will improve appropriate care as will the ability to offer services quickly in the acute phase.

Dr Joy Ratcliffe, Consultant in Old-Age Psychiatry, Manchester Mental Health and Social Care Trust

Older people have a higher rate of completed suicide than other age groups (World Health Organization 2002). Most elderly people who commit suicide are suffering from depression, and self-harm is greater in older depressed who have a poorly integrated social network and who feel hopeless (Dennis *et al.* 2005). The prevalence of hopelessness and suicidal ideation in older people has been reported to be between 0.7% and 17% and documentation of these ideas was noted in 38% of elderly who had committed suicide (Waern *et al.* 1999). Serious physical illness, particularly in men, is a risk factor for suicide in the elderly, with strong associations with visual impairment, neurological disorders and malignant disease (Waern *et al.* 2002).

The described case is of an older female with a history of depression who is the main carer of her husband with severe Parkinson's disease. She has depressive symptoms and reports that she can no longer go on and makes reference to 'mercy killing' to a practice nurse. It is unclear whether this is with regard to suicide, assisted suicide, a suicide pact, manslaughter or homicide. The National Institute for Clinical Excellence (2004b) recommend all self-harm in older people should be taken as suicide intent until proven otherwise. Further exploration is essential on what she meant by 'mercy killings', perhaps first by the practice nurse with involvement of the GP. This would be step 1 in stepped care described in the NICE Guidelines on depression (2004a). There should be a low threshold for involving mental health services which is likely to be to old-age psychiatry services (step 4 care). However there may be services for older people in the primary care mental health team (step 2 and 3 care), self-harm team or crisis intervention team. Secondary care services may have a self-harm team but may not accept referrals of the elderly and may not have staff with specific experience of self-harm in the elderly which NICE (2004b) recommends they should have. A survey of London Accident and Emergency psychiatry services found 66% accepted referrals of older people (Kewley and Bolton 2006). Excluding the elderly is age discriminatory and against Standard One of the National Service Framework for Older People (Department of Health 2001). Which service to refer her to would depend on what she meant by 'mercy killing' and local referral pathways in to each step of care. There may POVA (Protection Of Vulnerable Adults) issues with a duty to disclose information to social services if she had thoughts of harming/killing her husband.

To assess the risk of suicide questioning needs to start with exploring ideas of hopelessness and despair, thoughts of life not being worth living, a passive wish to die, suicidal ideation, suicidal plans and suicide attempts. Fears and stigma may lead to people masking suicidal ideation.

Further assessment is needed on current and past mental health and the social situation. With regard to management, the first consideration will be to decide the setting, either in the community at home, day hospital, intermediate care or whether she will need psychiatric in-patient care (step 5 care), either informal or by detention under the Mental Health Act 1983. With regard to treatment with antidepressants, selective serotonin reuptake inhibitors (SSRIs) are now widely accepted as the first-line choice in the treatment of depression, particularly as they are less dangerous than tricyclic antidepressants if taken in overdose. However this would need balancing against the increased risk of SSRIs causing gastrointestinal bleeding, particularly in older people with additional risk for those taking drugs such as non-steroidal anti-inflammatory drugs (NSAIDs) (Paton and Ferrier 2005). Psychological therapy will be needed to address depression and loss or bereavement issues. Such therapies are not always readily available for elderly people, although provision in the voluntary sector agencies should be explored.

Consideration will need to be given to support her husband with his Parkinson's disease including the identification of roles and responsibilities of the social worker (for home care, day care, respite, aids and adaptations), a Parkinson's disease nurse specialist, active case manager, physiotherapist, occupational therapist and palliative care team (NICE 2006).

Collaborative working would be improved with the Single Assessment Process (SAP) (Department of Health 2002), clear service pathways with a single point of entry and integration of health and social services, perhaps with the same computer system.

Case 5.3 Depression and forgetfulness

Miss Lucy R, 83 years old, lives in a flat near to her niece, Margaret. For the last six months, Margaret has noticed that Lucy has not been eating the food that they buy together when they go shopping once a week. Miss LR seems forgetful and more irritable than usual and her niece is worried that she is losing weight. Miss LR has stopped going to her local library because she says it has moved and she can't find it. Occasionally Miss LR has been upset when she is told that she has forgotten something and last week she shouted at Margaret and told her not to come again, something which the niece thought was quite out of character for her aunt. Yesterday she shouted at Margaret 'Go away and leave me alone, you don't care about me', and she burst into tears.

Miss LR has been reasonably well apart from hypertension (she has taken bendrofluazide for years). She has never married and always been regarded as being 'timid' by her family, but had always been close to her niece, particularly since the death of Miss LR's sister (Margaret's mother) 15 years ago, when Margaret recalls Miss LR became withdrawn and upset for a few months. Miss LR used to be house-proud but Margaret has noticed that the house smells of urine and she is not sure if this is due to Miss LR being incontinent (she dare not broach the subject with her aunt) or whether it is one of the three cats.

What is the likelihood of this being a mood disorder? How can Miss LR's apparent reluctance to accept help be addressed? What would be the management of this lady?

Professor Steve Iliffe, General Practitioner and Professor of Primary Care, Royal Free and University College Medical School, London
The working diagnosis for Miss LR is a depressive disorder within an early dementia syndrome, possibly with a complicating problem of urinary incontinence of unknown cause.

Depression is suggested by the three symptoms of reduced eating, weight loss and irritability. Of course these may be symptoms of a physical pathology too, so in investigating her further I would want to think about that possibility. She has an apparent history of a bereavement reaction that might predispose her to later depressive episodes, but her history is incomplete and needs further clarification.

Although depression can disrupt memory, the account of her not finding the local library and her uncharacteristic anger when her memory loss is pointed out could be features of an early dementia syndrome.

The niece has noticed that Miss LR's home smells of urine, but is unsure if this is due to the cats or Miss LR herself. If it is due to the cats, this level of neglect of the home is uncharacteristic for the house-proud Miss LR, and could fit with either a depressive disorder or a dementia syndrome. Urinary incontinence in Miss LR herself is unlikely to be attributable to the commonest forms of dementia, at least in the early stages, and needs further investigation.

We have no reason to think that Miss LR is reluctant to accept help, only that she reacts angrily when confronted about her memory loss. The task here is to gain and retain her trust, in sorting out her complex and potentially interwoven problems. This is something that the GP or practice nurse may be best placed to do, especially if they have developed a good enough working relationship with Miss LR over the years.

The first step is to review her medical records and discuss her with other practice staff who know her, particularly the practice nurse who is most likely to be managing Miss LR's hypertension, or reception staff who see her at the desk. Changes in Miss LR noticed by the nurse in recent months or even years may help identify subtle alterations in cognitive function, behaviour or functional ability that were insufficient to cause clinical concern at the time, but which in retrospect may have significance. The repeat medication record needs to be checked, to see if Miss LR has been ordering her prescriptions regularly; changes in medication use in older patients who are otherwise careful organizers of their own treatment are an early warning sign of cognitive impairment. A past history of depressive episodes may be important because this would increase her risks of a depressive disorder in later life.

The second step is to talk with Miss LR's niece. This situation is serious enough for your duty of care to override the duty of confidentiality, and the niece can provide important information about the pre-history of this problem. I would want to know about any changes in thinking, behaviour or mood in Miss LR over the two to three years prior to her situation becoming problematic. In particular I would want to learn about the extent to which the niece compensates for Miss LR's loss of abilities. For example, does she not only order the repeat medicines regularly, giving the GP the impression of orderly self-care, but also ensure that they are taken each day? Similarly, the niece may be able to describe the range of cognitive changes that could add up to a presumptive diagnosis of dementia syndrome. Finally, it may be necessary to agree with the niece how best to approach Miss LR and how best to respond to her. Direct challenges to her about her memory losses may not be productive, but continuing support will be, so some brief and mutual counselling at this stage could be useful.

The third step is to talk with Miss LR about her situation. This should be done in the first instance by the professional who knows her best, and in whom she has trust. This may be the practice nurse, or her usual GP. The management of her hypertension is the opportunity to talk with her about her health, and I would use the SPICE heuristic (Senses, Physical abilities, Incontinence, Cognition, Emotion) to structure that discussion (Iliffe *et al.* 2004). This is a helpful way to review possible co-morbidities like visual function loss or increasingly painful arthritis that may complicate her situation and compound the effects of any cognitive decline. Routine blood tests for hypertension management can be supplemented with a full blood count, erythrocyte sedimentation rate and C-reactive protein (as screens for other pathologies), glucose, thyroid function and calcium levels, to construct a dementia workup. Checking her weight may show that the niece is right, and open the discussion about appetite, energy and mood. Urine analysis is needed to exclude an occult urinary tract infection.

Making the diagnosis of dementia syndrome in general practice is a stepwise process and there is no reason to attempt to obtain all necessary information in one encounter. It is essential, however, to organize several consultations, making the maintenance of trust the first priority in all meetings with Miss LR. The clinical tasks can be passed from practice nurse to GP, with Miss LR's agreement, and when appropriate, but all professionals need to be assessing the severity of any depression symptoms, estimating the extent of cognitive losses and gaining some sense of Miss LR's capacity to make decisions. Ascertaining the number, severity and duration of depressive symptoms will help to categorize Miss LR's apparent depression, and can help guide decisions about which treatment to offer.

It is useful to measure both depression symptoms and cognitive function, so I would favour using the Mini-Mental Status Examination (MMSE) or the 6-item Cognitive Impairment Test (6-CIT), and the 15-item version of the Geriatric Depression Scale (GDS), if Miss LR is willing to allow this (see Chapter 7). With or without these measures, a picture of Miss LR's health status will emerge, and the initial diagnosis will be confirmed, modified or challenged.

If she does appear to have a depressive disorder superimposed on the early stages of a dementia syndrome, and she agrees with my view of what is happening to her, she should be offered treatment for both. The Royal College of Psychiatrists' guidelines help to frame psychological and medication treatment options in late-life depression (Baldwin *et al.* 2003), although psychological interventions will depend on local resources. The dementia syndrome needs specialist reassessment both to confirm my suspicions and to sub-type the dementia with a view to active treatment with cholinesterase inhibitors if she has a predominantly Alzheimer-type dementia (NICE/SCIE 2006) so the engagement of an old-age psychiatrist is the fourth step. This may at first be a telephone discussion rather than a formal referral, but at some stage a meeting between the specialist and Miss LR will be needed, in her home or at an outpatient clinic.

The fifth step is to set up the systematic follow-up for Miss LR and her niece, which will be needed whether or not shared care of drug treatment is undertaken. Both Miss LR and her niece will have to adjust to the diagnoses that have been made, antidepressant therapy will need to be monitored, and simple supportive counselling should given to both (in addition to any more complex psychological therapies offered).

Throughout the management of this lady, the GP needs to remain the key point of contact for the niece and collaborate effectively with other primary care and secondary care colleagues.

Professor Cornelius Katona, Dean, and Dr Chris Fox, Consultant and Senior Lecturer in Psychiatry, Kent Institute of Medicine and Health Sciences, University of Kent
Miss LR's most prominent presenting problem is her self-neglect as reflected in her reduced food intake and dirty, smelly and neglected home environment. It is also clear from the information given that she has become forgetful and that there are also prominent features suggestive of mood disturbance such as irritability and tearfulness. Given that there is no previous history of psychiatric disorder except for some distress following her sister's death (which appears to have been a normal grief reaction) the presentation with a

six-month history of functional decline and fluctuating mood makes a primary mood disorder unlikely.

A dementia syndrome is much more likely. The history of hypertension increases the possibility of a vascular aetiology to such a syndrome and would also increase the vulnerability to prominent affective symptoms. It must be added that depressive symptoms are also not uncommon in people with mild or moderate Alzheimer's disease (and indeed those with other dementias such as dementia with Lewy bodies (DLB), fronto-temporal dementia (FTD) and the dementia of Parkinson's disease (PDD). Long-term alcohol abuse should also be considered as a possible cause of cognitive decline; some older people are very adept at concealing their excessive drinking and indirect evidence (such as bin-loads of empty bottles) may be indicative. Verbal aggression is common in people with dementia and may be particularly distressing to relatives. These features may all be considered within the umbrella of the behavioural and psychological symptoms of dementia (BPSD).

Older people (particularly those with pre-existing cognitive deterioration of whatever cause) are vulnerable to acute confusion in the context of physical illness such as urinary or respiratory tract infection or after myocardial infarction or stroke. Occult malignancy may rarely present with confusion, usually related to elevated calcium levels. In Miss LR's case, the smell of urine raises the specific possibility of a urinary tract infection. Such infections are often clinically silent in older people (so symptoms such as dysuria and frequency may be absent or unnoticed). Given her use of a diuretic (which may have been taken erratically or excessively) electrolyte disturbance may also be contributing to her cognitive decline. Poor food intake and consequent hypoglycaemia may aggravate such confusion further. Persecutory ideas (and verbal or even physical aggression) are common features of acute confusional (delirious) states.

A physical examination will be helpful in identifying possible causes of delirium (such as fever, or the chest signs of a respiratory infection) and focal neurological signs which might suggest past or recent stroke. The presence of fever, reduced skin turgor and abnormalities of pulse or blood pressure would also be informative in this regard.

First-line investigations, which should be carried out in primary care, have been described by Steve Iliffe (see previous section). Other occasionally informative blood screening tests include syphilis serology and B_{12} and folate levels. Elevated erythrocyte sedimentation rate, C-reactive protein or plasma viscosity may suggest infection, malignancy or autoimmune disease (a rarer cause of cognitive decline). Urine culture and microscopy and an electrocardiogram are also first-line screening investigations and a chest X-ray is indicated if there is any specific suggestion of chest disease.

Risk assessment takes equal priority with diagnostic investigation. Key questions include evidence of physical consequences of neglect; confusion-related vulnerability (getting lost); being abused (by strangers or even carers); impaired driving skills; reduced road sense; inability to manage financial affairs; and risk of deliberate self-harm in the context of fluctuating low mood. Psychosocial assessment will also be crucial both in establishing a diagnosis and in formulating a management plan. Key questions include assessment of daily living skills (including food preparation and hygiene) and social support networks. These aspects of the assessment can usually be completed by most members of multi-professional old-age psychiatry teams.

Many teams find it useful to incorporate standardized rating scales into their assessments of people with mood disorders and cognitive impairment. Examples of such tests include the Mini-Mental State Examination (cognition), the Bristol Assessment of Daily Living Scale (BADL) and the Geriatric Depression Scale for mood (see Chapter 7).

The information collected above should be helpful in formulating an initial management plan which can best be developed thorough multi-professional team discussion. It may at this stage be possible to reach a firm diagnosis but further (second-line) investigation such as neuro-imaging (computer tomography (CT) or magnetic resonance imaging (MRI) scanning) may be necessary. Other key components in a management plan will include engaging the patient and carer; treating any acute condition found (such as an infection) and taking appropriate steps to reduce risk. Simple measures such as home-care input, electronic alarms and provision of regular meals may suffice. People with dementia at substantial risk (for example of harm through self-neglect, vulnerability to abuse, or self-harm) may need voluntary or compulsory placement in residential, nursing or hospital facilities. If this proved necessary for Miss LR, effective teamwork and communication with her and with her niece as well as with the primary care team will be crucial.

Specific medical and psychosocial interventions may be helpful to Miss LR, depending on the diagnosis reached. If she has moderate Alzheimer's disease, cholinesterase inhibitors may be helpful. In more severe disease (and possibly in the context of agitation) memantine (now subject to prescribing restrictions in England) may also be helpful. If she has a vascular dementia, consideration should be given to reducing vascular risk factors (by optimizing blood pressure control or giving anti-platelet agents). BPSD symptoms may respond to anti-psychotics though these must be used with great care in people like Miss LR in the light of the possibly increased risk of stroke, glucose dysregulation or further cognitive decline. The risk is greater still in people with DLB and PDD. Prominent depressive symptoms (and associated agitation) may respond to antidepressants, though several studies suggest that spontaneous remission often occurs and the placebo response rate is high. Monitoring progress following initiation of drug treatment will, ideally, be shared between the primary and secondary care teams. Cognitive decline may be slowed by intensive psychological interventions (e.g. cognitive stimulation) and BPSD symptoms can be responsive to focussed behavioural interventions which may also be of direct benefit to carers. Provision of such interventions depends on availability of appropriately trained staff. It is vital that the GP remains involved in the care of this more complex patient, even though decision-making may seem to be in the secondary care old-age community mental health team.

Editors' comments

We feel that the case commentaries illustrate the following important points.

Notes on Case 5.1

- The GP's prior knowledge of a patient can be vital in the detection of changes in a patient's mood and in the engagement and management of a patient with depression.
- Disordered thoughts and auditory hallucinations are features of psychotic depression.
- An assessment of risk to patient and risks to others is vital when psychotic depression is suspected.
- An assessment under the Mental Health Act may be appropriate in cases such as this.
- An urgent specialist mental health assessment should be requested when significant risk to self or others is demonstrated.
- Psychotic depression may be one of the indications for ECT.
- Collaboration between primary and secondary care professionals will be vital to manage a patient with psychotic depression at home.
- Concordance with medication can be improved by the use of appropriate packaging.

Notes on Case 5.2

- An awareness of the risk factors for suicide is vital to ensure risk is explored in all patients presenting with depression.
- NICE (2004b) recommend all self-harm in older people should be taken as suicide intent until proven otherwise.
- Initial prescriptions should be 7 to 14 days when there are thoughts of self-harm.
- Referral to step 4 (specialist mental health services) will be required if there is suicidal intent.
- A single point of access to specialist mental health services is desirable.

Notes on Case 5.3

- Depression can present with memory loss ('pseudo-dementia'), but early dementia can present with low mood and poor concentration which mimics depression.
- A history from formal and informal carers can be helpful – but beware of breaches in confidentiality.
- Several consultations may be needed to unravel complex cases such as this.
- Physical examination and investigation will exclude new physical pathology, or monitor known co-morbidity.
- Assessment of cognitive function should include the MMSE or equivalent.
- Specialist referral may be required to obtain a definitive diagnosis.
- Where dementia is suspected a different range of risks compared to depressive disorder should be addressed. These include self-neglect, personal safety and exploitation.
- Primary, secondary and social care must work together to achieve optimum management of patients with complex problems.

REFERENCES

Baldwin R., Anderson D., Block S., *et al.* (2003) Guidelines for the management of late-life depression in primary care. *Int. J. Geriatr. Psychiatry* **18**, 829–38.

Chantal, S., Everitt, H., Kendrick, T. (2005) *Oxford Handbook of General Practice.* Oxford, UK: Oxford University Press.

Dennis M., Wakefield P., Molloy C., Andrews H., Friedman T. (2005) Self-harm in older people with depression: comparison of social factors, life events and symptoms. *Br. J. Psychiatry* **186**, 538–9.

Department of Health (2001) *National Service Framework for Older People.* London: HMSO.

Department of Health (2002) *Guidance on the Single Assessment Process for Older People,* HSC2002/001: LAC (2002)1. London: HMSO.

Iliffe S., Lenihan P., Orrell M., *et al.* and the SPICE Research Team (2004) Involving the public in changing clinical practice: the development of a short instrument to identify common unmet needs in older people in general practice. *Br. J. Gen. Practice* **54**, 914–18.

Kewley T., Bolton J. (2006) A survey of liaison psychiatry services in general hospitals and accident and emergency departments: do we have the balance right? *Psychiatr. Bull.*, **30**, 260–3.

MHRA (2005) *Committee on Safety of Medicines Advice on Atypical Antipsychotics and Stroke.* London: Medicines and Healthcare Products Regulatory Agency. Available online at www.mhra.gov.uk/home/

NICE (2004a) *Depression: Management of Depression in Primary and Secondary Care,* Clinical Guideline No. 23. London: National Institute for Health and Clinical Excellence. Available online at www.nice.org.uk.

NICE (2004b) *Self-Harm: The Short-Term Physical and Psychological Management and Secondary Prevention of Self-Harm in Primary and Secondary Care*, Clinical Guideline No.16. London: National Institute for Health and Clinical Excellence. Available online at www.nice.org.uk.

NICE (2006) *Parkinson's Disease: Diagnosis and Management in Primary and Secondary Care*, Clinical Guideline No.35. London: National Institute for Health and Clinical Excellence. Available online at www.nice.org.uk.

NICE/SCIE (2006) *Dementia: The Treatment and Care of People with Dementia in Health and Social Care*, Clinical Guideline No. 42. London: National Institute for Health and Clinical Excellence/Social Care Institute for Excellence. Available online at www.nice.org.uk.

Paton C., Ferrier I. (2005) SSRIs and gastrointestinal bleeding. *Br. Med. J.*, **331**, 529–30.

Waern M., Beskow J., Runeson B., Skoog I. (1999) Suicidal feelings in the last year of life in elderly people who commit suicide. *Lancet*, **354**, 917–18.

Waern M., Rubenowitz E., Runeson B., *et al.* (2002) Burden of illness and suicide in elderly people: case-control study. *Br. Med. J.*, **324**, 1355–7.

World Health Organization (2002) *Suicide Prevention*. Available online at www.who.int/mental_health/prevention/suicide.

6

Management of late-life depression around the world: summary of international commentaries

International commentaries for the integrated management of depression

We asked clinicians from different countries to comment on the case history below, wherever possible as a joint response from a primary care physician and a specialist in psychiatry.

Case 6.1 Breathlessness and irritability

Miss Laura C is an 82-year-old lady with severe osteoarthritis and chronic obstructive pulmonary disease. She stopped smoking in her 60s and is very resentful that her breathlessness is so troublesome. She gets so much pain in her back and knees that she doesn't always feel like going down to the communal room in her sheltered (warden-supervised) accommodation or to the weekly lunch at the local church group.

Miss LC feels that her sleep is affected by her shortness of breath and the pain in her knees, and she has been waking in the early hours of the morning and not getting back to sleep. She feels tired, irritable and miserable all the next day and tends to nap every afternoon. She knows that people have called on her or have telephoned, but she admits that she often cannot bother to answer. She feels very lonely and over the past month has wondered if life is worth living.

The following synopsis encompasses contributions from Australia, Bulgaria, Canada, Denmark, France, Hong Kong, Japan, The Netherlands, Norway, Romania, Spain and the USA (see List of Contributors). The individual commentaries can be found in the Appendix.

Integrated Management of Depression in the Elderly, ed. C. Chew-Graham, R. Baldwin and A. Burns. Published by Cambridge University Press. © Cambridge University Press 2008.

Health-care systems

Most countries have a national health-care system under which Miss LC would be treated, usually accessed via a general practitioner (GP) or primary care physician (PCP). Countries differ as to whether provision comes from state funding, medical insurance, private health-care provision or a mixture. In Australia, private health-care among older people is uncommon (less than a third). In Denmark there is universal health coverage but medication is only 75% reimbursed which Abelskov and Christensen note can affect treatment concordance. In France patients can access specialists directly but without full reimbursement. Although access to specialists in France is likely to be more structured in the future, Robert and colleagues comment that a dual system may suit some older people as it offers more flexibility about where to seek care. The Hong Kong specialist psychiatric sector mirrors that of the UK but 'doctor-shopping' in the primary care sector is still common as the concept of 'family doctor' is still relatively new. Primary care provision may come from a PCP certificated in family medicine; one of the sizeable number of doctors who have not yet undergone vocational training in family medicine; or a non-primary care doctor providing primary care services in private practice, for example a general physician. In the Netherlands there is national GP coverage but for older people in nursing homes there are specially trained nursing home physicians with two years' postgraduate academic education. Norway has a three-tiered system for its national provision of health and social care based on the three interlinked national Acts. Local authorities manage a patient list system and each GP is responsible for a defined catchment area. The state runs the specialist services and hospitals. Private care is growing. Romania's system for mental health is largely hospital-based and psychiatrists are thinly spread – 4.16 per 100 000 of the population (currently a total of just under 22 million). Community care is however developing and the Mental Health Law 2002 has been a catalyst for reform of mental health services. Lyness and Campbell describe how the USA has no national health-care system and there are wide variations in practice due to factors such as state and local government policies (even regarding the implementation of federal programs such as Medicare and Medicaid).

Availability of specialist psychiatric services for older people is very variable. A consistent theme is scant resources in rural areas, away from major conurbations. For example in Australia, only the state of Victoria has well-established funded care for old-age psychiatry and Bulgaria has only 13 regional mental health centres from 28 administrative districts. Spain has a well-developed national health service: our Spanish contributors explained that that their unit was located in an urban health centre where specialists in family and community medicine work within a multidisciplinary team of nurses with a social worker and the support of the only unit for psychogeriatrics in Galicia, with monthly visits from an old-age psychiatrist. This arrangement is, however, uncommon certainly in those countries represented by our contributors.

Despite these differences in health-care availability and funding, Miss LC would first present to a GP (PCP) in most countries. The involvement by other specialists, for example physician or geriatrician, varied and was usually coordinated by the GP (PCP).

The presentation of depression

We asked our international contributors whether Miss LC's presentation of depression was typical or frequent in their country. In societies as diverse as Canada, Denmark, France, Hong Kong, Japan, Norway, Romania, Spain and the USA, the answer was a definite 'Yes'. Aspects that made the presentation characteristic were somatic preoccupation, medical co-morbidity and the minimization of a complaint of depressed mood. This is consistent with the published research in this area (see Chapter 1) concerning somatization and low expression of depressed mood in late-life depression, emphasizing that this is a cross-cultural phenomenon.

In terms of causal factors, medical illness (recent and chronic), disability, frailty, chronic pain and sleep difficulties were commented upon but so too was social isolation. In Japan, Awata commented that older people live in their own homes rather than in an assisted living facility. Nevertheless, in Japan isolation still contributes to depression, often in women after losing the husband because the surviving spouse may experience a lack of communication with other family members.

Assessment

All contributors described the necessity of taking a history of symptoms, a social history, examination of the mental state, noting particularly aspects of risk such as suicide and self-neglect, an assessment of cognition (often with a screening test for dementia such as the Mini-Mental State Examination (MMSE) (Folstein *et al.* 1975) or the Abbreviated Mental Test Score (AMTS) (Jitapunkul *et al.* 1991)) and a focussed physical assessment. The latter is to assess relevant co-morbidities such as chronic obstructive pulmonary disease (COPD) and arthritis in Miss LC's case and also to look for possible underlying unrecognized physical factors. For example Licht-Strunk and Bremmer from the Netherlands comment that heart failure in someone like Miss LC can easily be overlooked and might be precipitated by the introduction of non-steroidal anti-inflammatory drugs (NSAIDs) for pain. Investigations such as blood testing were not suggested universally but when discussed, contributors suggested a check for anaemia, a biochemical profile and thyroid function. Most contributors described the need to assess Miss LC's level of physical functioning and degree of impairment in relation to activities of daily living using clinical judgement rather than structured rating instruments.

The assessment of suicide risk was commented on by all contributors, although no specific tool or rating instrument was mentioned. Reliance was on a clinical evaluation of risk. Licht-Strunk and Bremmer specifically mention previous attempts, agitation, impulsivity, psychotic symptoms and substance misuse as risk factors. All contributors advised the need for admission of patients at high risk to a specialist mental health facility.

The use of rating instruments fell into two categories: tests to screen for the presence of depression and those to rate its severity. The Geriatric Depression Scale (GDS) in its different versions was the most widely advocated (Denmark, France, Hong Kong, Romania, Spain) for use in primary care (see Chapter 7). Of the severity measures, the Hamilton Rating Scale for Depression (HAM-D) and the Montgomery Asberg Depression Scale (MADRAS) (both outlined in Chapter 7) were advocated but their use was largely confined to specialist practice. Chiu and colleagues from Hong Kong mention that the GDS, HAM-D and the AMTS have all been translated into local languages and have some local validation data. Incentives to use some of these scales exist in some countries, for example Denmark and Norway. In the latter, the MADRAS score may determine management: between 16 and 35 indicates the need for a discussion with the patient about initiating antidepressant treatment and above 35 an immediate referral to the local specialist mental health service.

Awata from Japan strongly advocates that primary care physicians use a brief scale for depressive disorders to assess symptom severity, risk of suicide, and health-related quality of life of elderly depressed patients. Recommended is the WHO-Five Well-Being Index (WHO-5) (World Health Organization 2005). Since each item concerns positive well-being, health-care professionals are willing to use it and elderly community residents are likely to accept it. Awata comments that the scale has been translated into various languages and validated in the context of various psychiatric conditions including depressive disorders (Bonsignore *et al.* 2001, Henkel *et al.* 2003, 2004). It has good psychometric properties in older depressed patients (Heun *et al.*, 1999). Bonsignore *et al.* (2001) reported that the second version of the WHO-5 performs well in detecting depressive disorders in elderly primary care patients. Awata also suggests that the WHO-5 might be helpful for preventing suicide through improved patient management of depression (Hegerl and Althaus 2003). The Japanese version of the WHO-5 has also been validated in the context of detecting depressive disorders in diabetic patients (Awata *et al.* 2007a) and suicidal ideation in the general elderly population (Awata *et al.* 2007b).

In the USA, Campbell and Lyness discuss the Patient Health Questionnaire (PHQ-9) which is the tool advocated for use in primary care although not universally adopted. It is used both as a diagnostic aide and in monitoring treatment and its use is outlined further in Chapter 7.

Management

The commentators all agreed that optimizing medical care, reducing disability and handicap as far as possible, providing education about depression and encouraging social engagement are important first steps in management, with the GP (PCP) usually responsible for these. In Canada this co-ordinating role can be undertaken, following GP referral, by a Community Care Access Centre (CCAC) (see Ontario Ministry of Health 2007) which can mobilize a number of health-care professionals including PCPs, nurses, social workers and psychiatrists. These individuals or services can address the question of diagnosis of major depression as well as its management and monitor the response of other chronic illnesses to therapy. A recommendation of admission to a day programme may result.

Implicit in planning treatment is that the patient is informed and in agreement with the diagnosis, patient information leaflets are available in some countries (an example is given in Figure 6.1). According to Dutch law Miss LC will have to be informed about the diagnosis, her treatment options and possible harmful effects and she will have to consent to the treatment protocol.

When it comes to prescribing in primary care in every country the selective serotonin reuptake inhibitors (SSRIs) were mentioned as first-line treatments for a patient like Miss LC. Other first-line drugs were serotonin/noradrenaline reuptake inhibitors (SNRIs) (Canada, France, Romania, USA), moclobemide (France), noradrenaline and specific serotonin enhancers (NaSSa, mirtazepine) (Canada), bupropion (Canada) and mianserin (Norway). Second-line drugs (if the first was not effective or poorly tolerated) were: SNRIs (Bulgaria, Denmark, Hong Kong, Norway); NaSSa/mirtazepine (Bulgaria, Denmark, Norway); buspirone (Bulgaria); and noradrenaline reuptake inhibitors (NaRIs such as reboxetine) (Norway, Romania). Robert and colleagues from France and Ferreiro and Matteos from Spain recommend more activating antidepressants if apathy is present, mentioning fluoxetine, an SNRI or moclobemide. Tricyclic antidepressants were mentioned only as second-line drugs in severe depression (Bulgaria, Denmark, the Netherlands). Lithium augmentation of antidepressant treatment was virtually always initiated by specialist services although in Denmark the ongoing monitoring was by the GP.

Active follow-up was mentioned by our contributors from Denmark, France, the Netherlands and Norway, with an emphasis on medication maintenance for at least six months, usually coordinated by the GP (PCP).

All commentators recommended psychological interventions in addition to medication, although these were rarely available in primary care and only sporadically so in specialist services. The most commonly mentioned specific psychological intervention was cognitive behavioural therapy (CBT)

(Australia, Bulgaria, France, Hong Kong). In Australia, access to CBT is very limited due to the small number of practitioners available and willing to work with older people (Professor Ames writes that his local old-age psychiatry service does not at present employ a clinical psychologist with expertise in CBT), but new reimbursement regulations made in 2006 by the Australian federal government budget now permit the direct referral by GPs of patients to private clinical psychologists for a limited number of treatment sessions, the cost of which will be now be covered by the national universal health insurance scheme, Medicare. Ames and Flynn comment that it is likely that there will be steady growth in the use of CBT to treat depressions such as in Miss LC's case in future years. In the Netherlands, inter-personal therapy (IPT), another evidenced-based non-pharmacological intervention, would be recommended for Miss LC if it was considered that her depression had arisen within a context of inter-personal difficulties such as a dispute (with a friend of family member), a role transition (independent housing to sheltered housing), grief or inter-personal deficits (social impoverishment). Since this is a manual-based psychotherapy, it can be given by both psychotherapists and trained nurses.

Other brief therapies are available in primary care in some countries. Examples include problem-solving treatment (PST) in Japan via an outreach nurse supported by a psychiatrist, and in Spain a specific primary care brief psychotherapy (Tizón 1996).

In Bulgaria, Aleksandrova describes how supportive psychotherapy is the main mode of psychological intervention, with an emphasis on showing interest, concern, empathy, encouragement and acceptance as well as tackling specific problems and helping direct the patient to relevant services. CBT, if available, would be practised at a pace slower than that for younger patients and often with a more active role for the therapist.

Our commentators discussed a number of less specific but still helpful non-pharmacological interventions. In Denmark, as elsewhere, psychological interventions are limited in availability but if Miss LC was admitted to hospital there would be an emphasis on physiotherapy and work carried out in a group setting. In Norway, behavioural activation would be encouraged. This encourages purposeful activity using a diary or schedule. Support for care-givers of those with depressive disorder was encouraged. In Denmark the relatives of depressed patients are given two leaflets. One is about how to talk to and deal with a depressed relative. Abelskov and Christensen comment that a very frequent mistake made by relatives is to ask the patient to deal with multiple tasks all at once. The depressed patient may not be able to finish any of the tasks when faced with this and their confidence is further dented. The leaflet advises relatives to give information in bite-sized, simple chunks. The second leaflet describes symptoms, treatments and myths about depression.

We did not specifically ask about electroconvulsive treatment (ECT) but it was mentioned by our contributors from Denmark, Hong Kong and the

Netherlands. It was used in specialized psychiatric care for patients with intractable depression or who present with acute risk of self-harm or imminent risk to health because of food, fluid or medication refusal.

Systems working together

In all countries specialist services are available to support primary care in managing depression. Most often this occurs after initial treatment failure, if the condition is complex (for example if dementia is suspected) or there is acute risk, as in self-harm. Arrangements for the initiation, delivery and organization of social care differed markedly from country to country and was dependent on how social care was funded.

Barriers to effective treatment of older depressed patients

All but one of our commentators cited a lack of recognition of depression in later life as the single most important barrier to its successful treatment. This is not simply a GP or PCP problem, as several contributors saw this as operating in families and society as a whole (with depression still seen as 'normal' in older age) or with cultural barriers such as stigma or shame playing an additional part. The exception was Canada where Shulman and Upshur remark that clinicians, including PCPs, are attuned to the possibility of depressive disorder to a much greater extent than used to be the case and that, if anything, there may be a tendency to over-diagnose depression especially when cognitive impairment is beginning. Similarly, several contributors wrote that training delivered to GPs/PCPs in mental health has undoubtedly improved over the years.

The second most frequently cited barrier to effective management was a lack of psychological interventions. A lack of training opportunities in specific therapies such as CBT added to this problem. Our Australian and Canadian contributors saw low referral rates from primary to specialist services as another barrier. Ames from Australia demonstrates the problem. His old-age psychiatry service, covering 45 000 individuals aged above 65, receives approximately 700 new referrals for assessment each year. Yet taking a very conservative estimate of 1% of the elderly being affected by a major depressive disorder, he would expect there to be at least 450 old people with major depression within that catchment area at any given time, with a significant turnover of incident and recovering cases (even though many may be chronic). As the bulk of referrals to him are for people with dementia and disturbed behaviour, and a large proportion of the remaining referrals are for people with schizophrenia and related disorders, clearly the majority of elderly individuals with major depression are not being referred, despite the fact that his catchment has one of the most active, engaged community old-age psychiatry services in Australia. A caveat though is that in Hong Kong a major barrier is the long waiting times to see public sector specialist psychiatric services and in Spain too there are pressures on specialist services.

The third most frequently cited barrier was a lack of governmental investment, often in the face of competing demands. For example, in Hong Kong Chiu reports that the emphasis has shifted away from mental health toward concerns about infectious diseases such as avian influenza. Sadly, ageism may be implicated too – Endegal and Sanakar from Norway comment that resources may be prioritized to younger adults. In Romania a lack of investment in community resources was seen as a specific barrier to the care of older people with depression. Lastly, in the USA, the pioneering of new models of depression management (see below) is held up by a lack of funding for them.

Other barriers were mentioned. In Canada, a lack of outreach services to the community to counter isolation, important in Miss LC's case, was cited. In Denmark, medication costs may deter older adults from taking a recommended course of antidepressants and in the USA there may be funding issues too but additionally patients often refuse to take antidepressants. Also noted by our US contributors were difficulties in accessing services by particular ethnic groups. In Denmark, premature discontinuation of home care systems on the patient's say-so or if their mood seems to be improving was seen as a problem. So, even if after-care is available, as is it is in Denmark, a lack of education about depression among front-line workers may contribute to poor outcomes.

Protocols, guidelines and initiatives

Several of the initiatives described below are referenced in Chapter 7.

A number of sets of guidelines for the treatment of depression (most not focussed exclusively upon the elderly) have been developed by the Royal Australian College of GPs, the Royal Australian and New Zealand College of Psychiatrists and the government-funded public health depression initiative 'Beyond Blue' (www.beyondblue.org.au), and these can be consulted online. Ames and Flynn comment that it is fair to say that their utilization would be 'a custom more honoured in the breach than in the observance'. One initiative aimed at GPs examined the role of a multifaceted intervention to address mood disorder in a Sydney residential home complex, showing some evidence of modest, sustained benefit in the reduction of rates of depression among 1036 older residents (Llewellyn-Jones *et al.* 1999).

At the national level, the Canadian Network for Mood and Anxiety Treatments (Kennedy *et al.* 2001) has a well-organized approach to the management of patients with depressive and bipolar disorders (see also Chapter 7). These are available for individuals and professionals alike. CANMAT also provides help and resources specifically focussed on older adults including

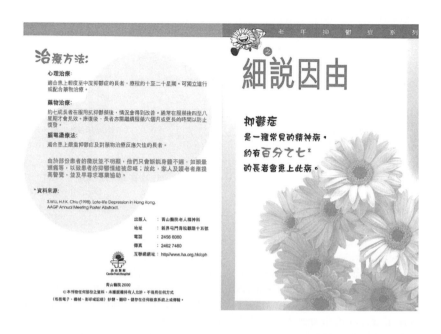

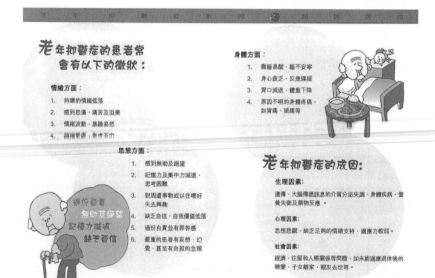

Figure 6.1 Example of a patient information leaflet.

explanations of contributing aetiological factors, risk factors (including for suicide) and a self-assessment guide using the GDS. CANMAT also focusses on the relationship between depression and a number of medical and neurological problems including hypothyroidism, Alzheimer's disease, Parkinson's disease, congestive heart failure and infectious diseases.

Shulman and Upshur also highlight an important new web-based resource 'Check Up from the Neck Up'. This website is a collaborative project of the Mood Disorders Association of Ontario and a number of other organizations including Sunnybrook Health Sciences Centre, University of Toronto where the Chief of Psychiatry, Dr Anthony Levitt, is an important resource for the website. This website provides self-assessment guidelines as well as a summary of available treatments including pharmacological and psychological approaches to the management of depression.

In May, 2006, the Canadian Coalition for Seniors' Mental Health (CCSMH) produced a comprehensive document entitled *National Guidelines for Seniors' Mental Health*. This coalition was established in 2002 following a conference hosted by the Canadian Academy of Geriatric Psychiatry. They established a guideline development group specifically for depression in older adults led by Dr Marie-France Tourigny Rivard of the University of Ottawa and Dr Diane Buchanan from the School of Nursing at Queen's University, Kingston, Ontario. These guidelines provide recommendations regarding screening and assessment for depression in older adults where specific risk factors are identified. Referring back to the case history, these factors include social isolation, chronic disabling illness, recent major physical illness (within three months), persistent sleep difficulties and significant somatic concerns, making Miss LC at significant risk for major depression. The guidelines suggest that following a positive screen for depression, a biopsychosocial assessment should be conducted to include a formal review of diagnostic criteria which in North American means the *Diagnostic and Statistical Manual* (DSM-IV) of the American Psychiatric Association (1994) or ICD-10 diagnostic manual (World Health Organization 1993). Also included are an estimate of the severity of depressive symptomatology, a specific risk assessment for suicide, a functional assessment, a review of personal and family history of mood disorder, a review of medication and substance abuse, a review of current stressors and life situation, supports available and personal strengths. In addition to the mental status examination, a formal cognitive screen is recommended, either the Mini-Mental State Examination or the Clock Drawing Test. More information about accessing the guidelines is given in Chapter 7.

The Japan Medical Association published *The Manual for Suicide Prevention* in 2004, which provides a guideline for PCPs in the diagnosis and treatment of depression. Also from Japan, Awata writes that an important nationwide social system to detect elderly depressed people in Japan is the community welfare volunteer, 'Minsei-iin', comprising individuals appointed in each community by the Minister of Health and Welfare for three-year terms. Their aim is to understand community needs and liaise with welfare offices and other community resources. Community welfare volunteers can be the first to identify distressed older people in which case they trigger a visit by a community nurse to evaluate depression and suicide risk.

In the Netherlands there are approximately 90 primary care guidelines for frequently met conditions and they are widely accepted and used. One is for depression and has wide uptake. It includes a list of the nine symptoms of depressive disorder according to DSM-IV and is used to screen for depression in high-risk groups.

In Australia and Spain local initiatives have been developed in collaboration with the pharmaceutical industry.

The USA has many national and regional guidelines for the management of depression in primary care, and while they are widely accepted in principle, in practice they are often not followed. Many physicians are starting to use the principles of chronic disease management or Wagner's Chronic Care Model to manage depression. These approaches include a multidisciplinary approach with treatment protocols, intensive patient education and follow-up and use of patient registries. Three quality measures for depression treatment have been widely accepted (including by HEDIS – Health plan Employer Data and Information Set, established by the National Committee for Quality Assurance) and are being tracked and reported by insurance companies. These include measuring the optimal clinician contact and follow-up of patients diagnosed with depression and whether patients stay on their antidepressant medications both acutely and chronically. Some insurance companies are starting to use these and other quality measures to rate physicians' clinical care and adjust their financial compensation, an approach called 'Pay for performance'. At the time of writing Medicare is about to begin such a program. It is expected, but yet to be demonstrated, that the inclusion of these depression quality measures in physician 'report cards' and pay-for-performance reimbursement systems will result in improvement in depression care. The USA has also pioneered the model of collaborative care in which PCPs and specialist services work together within a framework of agreed protocols to manage depression, with the care being co-ordinated by trained personnel, often a nurse. Lyness and Campbell highlight the strong evidence base showing that this model is effective in treating late-life depression in primary care (Unützer *et al.* 2002).

REFERENCES

American Psychiatric Association (1994) *Diagnostic and Statistical Manual,* Version IV. Washington, DC: APA.

Awata S., Bech P., Yoshida S., *et al.* (2007a) Reliability and validity of the Japanese version of the WHO-Five Well-Being Index in the context of detecting depression in diabetic patients. *Psychiatr. Clin. Neurosci.* **61**, 112–19.

Awata S., Bech P., Koizumi Y., *et al.* (2007b) Validity and utility of the Japanese version of the WHO-Five Well-Being Index in the context of detecting suicidal ideation in elderly community residents. *Int. Psychogeriatr.* **19**, 77–88.

Bonsignore M., Barkow K., Jessen F., Heun R. (2001) Validity of the five-item WHO Well-being index (WHO-5) in an elderly population. *Eur. Arch. Psychiatr. Clin. Neurosci.* **251**(Suppl. 2), II/27–II/31.

Canadian Coalition for Seniors' Mental Health (2006) *National Guidelines for Seniors' Mental Health: The Assessment and Treatment of Depression.* Available online at www.ccsmh.ca

Folstein M. F., Folstein S. E., McHugh P. R. (1975) 'Mini-Mental State': a practical method for grading the cognitive state of patients for the clinician. *J. Psychiatr. Res.* **12**, 185–98.

Hegerl U., Althaus D. (2003) From patient screening to management list in suicide risk: practical guidelines for dealing with depression. *MMW Fortshritte der Medizin* **145**, 24–27.

Henkel V., Mergl R., Kohnen R., *et al.* (2003) Identifying depression in primary care: a comparison of different methods in a prospective cohort study. *Br. Med. J.*, **326**, 200–1.

Henkel V., Mergl R., Coynbe J. C., *et al.* (2004) Screening for depression in primary care: will one or two items suffice? *Eur. Arch. Psychiatr. Clin. Neurosci.* **254**, 215–23.

Heun R., Burkart M., Maier M., Bech P. (1999) Internal and external validity of the WHO Well-Being Scale in the elderly general population. *Acta Psychiatr. Scand.* **99**, 171–8.

Japan Medical Association (2004) *The Manual for Suicide Prevention.* Tokyo: Japan Medical Association.

Jitapunkul S., Pillay I., Ebrahim S. (1991) The Abbreviated Mental Test: its use and validity. *Age Aging* **20**, 332–6.

Kennedy S. H., Lam R. W., and the CANMAT Depression Working Group (2001) Clinical guidelines for the treatment of depressive disorders. *Can. J. Psychiatry* **46**, (Suppl. 1), 1S–92S.

Llewellyn-Jones R., Baike K., Smithers H., Cohen J., Snowdon J. (1999) Multifaceted shared care intervention for late-life depression in residential care: randomized controlled trial. *Br. Med. J.* **319**, 676–82.

Ontario Ministry of Health (2007) *Community Care Access Centres.* Available online at www.health.gov.on.ca/english/public/contact/ccac/ccac_mn.html

Tizón J. L. *Componentes Psicológicos de la Práctica Médica: Una Perspectiva desde la Atención Primaria [Psychological Components of Medical Practice from the Primary Care Perspective]*, 4th edn. Barcelona: Doyma.

Unützer J., Katon W., Callahan C., *et al.* (2002) Collaborative care management of late-life depression in the primary care setting. *J. Am. Med. Assoc.* **288**, 2836–45.

World Health Organization (1993) *The ICD-10 Classification of Mental and Behavioural Disorders: Research Criteria.* Geneva: WHO.

World Health Organization (2005) *WHO-Five Well-Being Index.* Geneva: WHO. Availabel online at www.who-5.org

Resources

Robert Baldwin, Carolyn Chew-Graham and Alistair Burns

The aim of this chapter is bring together the variety of information found in the preceding chapters and commentaries into a practical resource for practitioners.

Screening for depression in older people

The usefulness of screening for depression depends on the baseline prevalence in the population screened; the higher the baseline prevalence the more likely is the screening to be cost-effective. Thus, targeted screening is more effective than screening an entire population. Examples include screening residents of a nursing home or the list of older patients on a general practice with physical conditions known to have strong links with depression, such as diabetes, chronic obstructive pulmonary disease or chronic heart disease (Krishnan et al. 2002). Iliffe and colleagues (page 95) add that screening should be linked to patients' perceptions of what is important and their SPICE acronym suggests five priority areas: senses, physical activity, incontinence, cognition and emotional distress.

The Geriatric Depression Scale (GDS) has been advocated as a screening instrument. It comprises 30 questions and takes about 10 minutes to complete (Table 7.1). The GDS avoids questions which rely on physical symptoms, and uses a simple yes/no format. Although designed to be self-administered, rater-assistance is acceptable. There are shorter versions, including a four-item (questions 1, 3, 8 and 9) and a 15-item version (Table 7.1) which may be more appropriate for use in primary care. There is a GDS website with the various versions, bibliography and translations into Chinese, Creole, Danish, Dutch, Farsi, French, French Canadian, German, Greek, Hebrew, Hindi, Hungarian, Icelandic, Italian, Japanese, Korean, Lithuanian, Malay, Portuguese, Russian, Russian Ukrainian, Spanish, Swedish, Thai, Turkish, Vietnamese and Yiddish (http://stanford.edu/~yesavage/GDS.html). In the UK, the GDS has been

Integrated Management of Depression in the Elderly, ed. C. Chew-Graham, R. Baldwin and A. Burns. Published by Cambridge University Press. © Cambridge University Press 2008.

Table 7.1 The Geriatric Depression Scale

Instructions: Choose the best answer for how you have felt over the past week.
 (1) **Are you basically satisfied with your life? No**
 (2) **Have you dropped many of your activities and interests? Yes**
 (3) **Do you feel your life is empty? Yes**
 (4) **Do you often get bored? Yes**
 (5) Are you hopeful about the future? No
 (6) Are you bothered by thoughts you can't get out of your head? Yes
 (7) **Are you in good spirits most of the time? No**
 (8) **Are you afraid something bad is going to happen to you? Yes**
 (9) **Do you feel happy most of the time? No**
 (10) **Do you often feel helpless? Yes**
 (11) Do you often get restless and fidgety? Yes
 (12) **Do you prefer to stay at home, rather than going out and doing new things? Yes**
 (13) Do you frequently worry about the future? Yes
 (14) **Do you feel you have more problems with your memory than most? Yes**
 (15) **Do you think it is wonderful to be alive now? No**
 (16) Do you often feel down-hearted and blue (sad)? Yes
 (17) **Do you feel pretty worthless the way you are? Yes**
 (18) Do you worry a lot about the past? Yes
 (19) Do you find life very exciting? No
 (20) Is it hard for you to start on new projects (plans)? Yes
 (21) **Do you feel full of energy? No**
 (22) **Do you feel that your situation is hopeless? Yes**
 (23) **Do you think most people are better off (in their lives) than you are? Yes**
 (24) Do you frequently get upset over little things? Yes
 (25) Do you frequently feel like crying? Yes
 (26) Do you have trouble concentrating? Yes
 (27) Do you enjoy getting up in the morning? No
 (28) Do you prefer to avoid social gatherings (get-togethers)? Yes
 (29) Is it easy for you to make decisions? No
 (30) Is your mind as clear as it used to be? No

Notes: (a) Answers refer to responses which score '1'; (b) bracketed phrases refer to alternative ways of expressing the questions; (c) questions in bold comprise the 15-item version.
Suggested meaning of scores (GDS-30):
    0–4: normal, depending on age, education, complaints
    5–8 mild
    8–11 moderate
    12–15 severe
Thresholds for a possible case of depression $\geq$5 for GDS-15 and $\geq$2 for GDS-4.

Table 7.2 The Caribbean Culture-Specific Screen for emotional distress

---

In the past month:
 (1) Have you been worrying too much or fretting?
 (2) Have you felt pressured, like pressure is rising in your head?
 (3) Have you had lots of pain or gas in the belly or the pit of your stomach?
 (4) What about pain or aching all over the body?
 (5) Have you felt weak or tired a lot of the time?
 (6) Have you slept well most of the time?
 (7) Have you been feeling down or low spirited or like you're crying inside?
 (8) Have you felt palpitations or fear around the heart?
 (9) Have you felt fed up with yourself or even with others, like you want to curse or scream?
 (10) Have you felt cut or alone, like people don't appreciate you?
 (11) Or been feeling empty or spiritless inside?
 (12) Do you feel weighed down by life?
 (13) Do you still feel hopeless?

Note: For all questions except (6), score 1 for 'yes'; for question (6) score 1 for 'no'. A score of ≥ 5 indicates a possible case of depression.

endorsed for use in primary care by the Royal College of General Practitioners (Williams and Wallace 1993).

In Chapter 1, Waheed discussed the GDS from a cross-cultural perspective. Studying an African-Caribbean community, Abas *et al.* (1998) found that for detecting clinical depression the GDS had good sensitivity and specificity at the recommended cut-off of >5 or =5 but a lower threshold of 4 was required if the more culturally delineated syndrome of 'depressed/lost spirit' was to be detected. Dr Rait and colleagues (1999) too recommended a GDS cut-off of ≥ 4, and Dr Waheed mentioned the Caribbean Culture-Specific Screen for emotional distress (CCSD). Although it performs no better than the GDS in African-Caribbean older people it is the only such culturally specific instrument and is therefore reproduced (Table 7.2).

The Patient Health Questionnaire (PHQ-9) (Table 7.3) can be used for both screening for depression in primary care and as a means of measuring severity (Table 7.4) (Kroenke *et al.* 2001). It scores each of the nine DSM-IV criteria (American Psychiatric Association 1994) from 0 (not at all) to 3 (nearly every day). For screening purposes one or both of the first two questions should score at least 2. For a more definite diagnosis of major depression, five or more questions must be rated as 2 or 3, except for question 9, for which any score above 0 is significant. In addition, question 10, functional impairment, is endorsed as at least 'somewhat difficult'. Detailed information about scoring can be found at www.depression-primarycare.org/about/mission/.

PATIENT HEALTH QUESTIONNAIRE (PHQ-9)

NAME: _____ DATE: _____

Over the *last 2 weeks*, how often have you been bothered by any of the following problems? (*use "✓" to indicate your answer*)	not at all	several days	more than half the days	nearly every day
1. Little interest or pleasure in doing things	0	1	2	3
2. Feeling down, depressed, or hopeless	0	1	2	3
3. Trouble falling or staying asleep, or sleeping too much	0	1	2	3
4. Feeling tired or having little energy	0	1	2	3
5. Poor appetite or overeating	0	1	2	3
6. Feeling bad about yourself – or that you are a failure or have let yourself or your family down	0	1	2	3
7. Trouble concentrating on things, such as reading the newspaper or watching television	0	1	2	3
8. Moving or speaking so slowly that other people could have noticed. Or the opposite – being so fidgety or restless that you have been moving around a lot more than usual	0	1	2	3
9. Thoughts that you would be better off dead, or of hurting yourself in some way	0	1	2	3
add columns:		+	+	+
TOTAL:				

(Healthcare professional: For interpretation of TOTAL, please refer to accomanying scoring card.)

10. If you checked off *any* problems, how *difficult* have these problems made it for you to do your work, take care of things at home, or get along with other people?

Not difficult at all ___
Somewhat difficult ___
Very difficult ___
Extremely difficult ___

Table 7.4 Suggested severity scales for the PHQ-9

PHQ-9 score	Provisional diagnosis	Treatment recommendation
5–9	Minimal symptoms	Support, educate to call if worse; return in 1 month
10–14	Minor depression Dysthymia Major depression, *mild*	Support, watchful waiting Antidepressant or psychotherapy Antidepressant or psychotherapy
15–19	Major depression, *moderately severe*	Antidepressant or psychotherapy
≥20	Major depression, *severe*	Antidepressant <u>and</u> psychotherapy (especially if not improved on monotherapy)

Source: PHQ-9 © 1999 Pfizer Inc. All rights reserved. Reproduced with permission.

The World Health Organization Well-Being Index was developed as a quick depression screen based on an older questionnaire (called the Zung Inventory). The 1998 version (version 2) is reproduced in Table 7.5 and has been validated on people aged 50 and above (Bonsignore *et al.* 2001). A higher score indicates greater well-being. A score below 13 or a score of 0 to 1 on any of the five items suggests a high likelihood of depressive disorder.

The Brief Assessment Schedule Depression Cards (BASDEC) (Adshead *et al.* 1992) is unusual in comprising a 19-item deck of cards requiring yes/no responses and has been translated into Bengali, Gujarati, Hindi, Punjabi and Urdu. It is useful where privacy is difficult. BASDEC is available for a small charge from www.basdec.co.uk/.

Although not emphasized in the commentaries, other scales include: the Beck Depression Inventory (Beck *et al.* 1961) which is copyrighted, Center for Epidemiologic Studies Depression Scale (CES-D) (Radloff 1977) and the SelfCARE(D) (Bird *et al.* 1987), both of which have been widely used in epidemiological research rather than everyday practice.

Cocksedge (page 90) lists the main risk factors for suicide in older people and suggests eight relevant questions. Rating scales of suicidal thinking exist but their use is not straightforward as there are concerns that the relatively detached administration of a questionnaire to someone who requires immense empathy may make matters worse. For those interested, these and other issues regarding suicide can be further explored on the website of the Canadian Coalition for Seniors' Mental Health (CCSMH) (www.ccsmh.ca) which has recently produced a downloadable guideline on the assessment of suicide risk and prevention of suicide in older people. For a general review of the performance of screening instruments in primary care, see Watson and Pigmore (2003).

Table 7.5 WHO-5 Well-Being Index (WHO-Five)

Please indicate for each of the five statements which is closest to how you have been feeling over the last two weeks. Notice that higher numbers mean better well-being. **Example: If you have felt cheerful and in good spirits more than half of the time during the last two weeks, put a tick in the box with the number 3 beside it.**

	All of the time	Most of the time	More than half of the time	Less than half of the time	Some of the time	At no time
(1) I have felt cheerful and in good spirits	☐ 5	☐ 4	☐ 3	☐ 2	☐ 1	☐ 0
(2) I have felt calm and relaxed	☐ 5	☐ 4	☐ 3	☐ 2	☐ 1	☐ 0
(3) I have felt active and vigorous	☐ 5	☐ 4	☐ 3	☐ 2	☐ 1	☐ 0
(4) I woke up feeling fresh and rested	☐ 5	☐ 4	☐ 3	☐ 2	☐ 1	☐ 0
(5) My daily life has been filled with things that interest me	☐ 5	☐ 4	☐ 3	☐ 2	☐ 1	☐ 0

The commentaries also illustrate the importance of screening for dementia in the older depressed person who may appear confused. The Mini-Mental Status Examination (MMSE) (Folstein *et al.* 1975) covers orientation, registration, attention, calculation and language and takes about 10 minutes. Its use is copyrighted (www.minimental.com/) but useful information can be found on the Alzheimer's Society website (www.alzheimers.org.uk) following the links How Dementia is Diagnosed and clicking on the MMSE fact sheet. A dementia tutorial which includes the MMSE can also be found on the Alzheimer's Society website by following the links: Working with People with Dementia – Primary Care – Resources for Primary Care and opening the file Dementia: Diagnosis and Management in Primary Care.

A shorter screening scale for dementia is the 6-item Orientation–Memory–Concentration (OMC) test (Katzman *et al.* 1983) (Table 7.6). A score of above 10 indicates likely significant confusion. Also called the 6-CIT, it has been compared to the MMSE by Brooke and Bullock (1999) who recommended some simplification of its scoring system with a redefined threshold score of 7/8. The clock-drawing test, also mentioned, is quite widely used. There are several scoring methods and these are discussed by Shulman (2000).

Table 7.6 Orientation–Memory–Concentration test (OMC)

Question No.		Maximum error	Score ×	Weight
(1)	What year is it now?	1	____ × 4	= ____
(2)	What month is it now?	1	____ × 3	= ____
	Repeat this phrase:			
	John Brown, 42 Market Street, Chicago			
	or (UK):			
	John Brown, 42 West Street, Gateshead			
(3)	About what time is it? (within 1 hour)	1	____ × 3	= ____
(4)	Count backwards 20 to 1	2	____ × 2	= ____
(5)	Say the months in reverse order	2	____ × 2	= ____
(6)	Repeat the phrase just given	5	____ × 2	= ____
			Total error score	= ___/28

Assessment of severity

The Hamilton Rating Scale for Depression (HAM-D) (Hamilton 1960) and the Montgomery Äsberg Depression Rating Scale (MADRAS) (Montgomery and Äsberg 1979) are mentioned by several commentators. They are reproduced respectively in Tables 7.7 and 7.8. The HRDS covers 17 items and is observer-rated and the MADRAS is a mixture of self-report and observed behaviour. A 50% reduction in either scale is regarded as a treatment 'response' and a remission as a score of <7 or <10 respectively. In their commentary Engedal and Sanaker suggest a MADRAS threshold of 36 and above for immediate referral to psychiatric services. Time restraints often limit the use of such scales in primary care, and the PHQ-9 severity scale may be a useful alternative (Table 7.4) and has the advantage that the severity score can be linked broadly to treatment strategies.

Colleagues from France mentioned evaluating apathy. Low motivation may be a particular feature of later-life depression and is a symptom not captured particularly well by current depression schedules. The Apathy Evaluation Scale Inventory (Marin *et al.* 1991) is used in specialist settings and more information can be found at www.tbims.org/combi/; click on the links to Scales and then the Apathy Evaluation Scale.

Practice guidelines (practitioner resources)

Treatment of depression

Alexopoulos and colleagues (Alexopoulos *et al.* 2001) have written an expert consensus document on the pharmacotherapy of late-life depression. The

Table 7.7 The Hamilton Rating Scale for Depression (HAM-D)

(1) DEPRESSED MOOD (sadness, hopeless, helpless, worthless)

    0 = Absent

    1 = These feeling states indicated only on questioning

    2 = These feeling states spontaneously reported verbally

    3 = Communicates feeling states non-verbally – i.e. through facial expression, posture, voice, and tendency to weep

    4 = Patients reports VIRTUALLY ONLY these feeling states in his spontaneous verbal and non-verbal communication

(2) FEELINGS OF GUILT

    0 = Absent

    1 = Self-reproach

    2 = Ideas of guilt or rumination over past errors or sinful deeds

    3 = Present illness is a punishment. Delusions of guilt

    4 = Hears accusatory or denunciatory voices and/or experiences threatening visual hallucinations

(3) SUICIDE

    0 = Absent

    1 = Feels life is not worth living

    2 = Wishes he were dead or any thoughts of possible death to self

    3 = Suicide ideas or gestures

    4 = Attempts at suicide (any serious attempts rates 4)

(4) INSOMNIA EARLY

    0 = No difficulty falling asleep

    1 = Complains of occasional difficulty falling asleep – ie. more than half an hour

    2 = Complains of nightly difficulty falling asleep

(5) INSOMNIA MIDDLE

    0 = No difficulty

    1 = Patient complains of being restless and disturbed during the night

    2 = Waking during the night – any getting out of bed rates 2 (except for the purposes of voiding)

(6) INSOMNIA LATE

    0 = No difficulty

    1 = Waking in early hours of the morning but goes back to sleep

    2 = Unable to fall asleep again if he gets out of bed

(7) WORK AND ACTIVITIES

    0 = No difficulties

    1 = Thoughts and feelings of incapacity, fatigue or weakness related to activities; work or hobbies

    2 = Loss of interest in activity; hobbies or work – either directly reported by patient, or indirect in listlessness, indecision and vacillation (feels he has to push self to work or activities)

    3 = Decrease in actual time spent in activities or decrease in productivity. In hospital rate 3 if patient does not spend at least 3 hours a day in activities (hospital job or hobbies) exclusive of ward chores

Table 7.7 (*cont.*)

4 = Stopped working because of present illness. In hospital, rate 4 if patient engages in no activities except ward chores, or if patient fails to perform ward chores unassisted

(8) RETARDATION

0 = Normal speech and thought

1 = Slight retardation at interview

2 = Obvious retardation at interview

3 = Interview difficult

4 = Complete stupor

(9) AGITATION

0 = None

1 = Fidgetiness

2 = Playing with hands, hair, etc.

3 = Moving about, can't sit still

4 = Hand wringing, nail biting, hair pulling, biting of lips

(10) ANXIETY: PSYCHIC

0 = No difficulty

1 = Subjective tension and irritability

2 = Worrying about minor matters

3 = Apprehensive attitude apparent in face or speech

4 = Fears expressed without questioning

(11) ANXIETY: SOMATIC

0 = Absent

Psychological concomitants of anxiety such as:

1 = Mild gastrointestinal – dry mouth, wind, indigestion, diarrhoea

2 = Moderate cramps, belching

3 = Severe cardiovascular – palpitations, headaches

4 = Incapacitating respiratory – hyperventilation, sighing, urinary frequency, sweating

(12) SOMATIC SYMPTOMS: GASTROINTESTINAL

0 = None

1 = Loss of appetite but eating without staff encouragement. Heavy feeling in abdomen

2 = Difficulty eating without staff urging. Requests or requires laxatives or medication for bowels or medication for gastrointestinal symptoms

(13) SOMATIC SYMPTOMS: GENERAL

0 = None

1 = Heaviness in limbs, back or head. Backaches, headache, muscle aches. Low energy and fatiguability

2 = Any clear-cut symptoms rates 2

(14) GENITAL SYMPTOMS

0 = Absent

1 = Mild symptoms such as: loss of libido, menstrual disturbances

2 = Severe symptoms

Table 7.7 (*cont.*)

---

(15) HYPOCHONDRIASIS
    0 = Not present
    1 = Self-absorption (bodily)
    2 = Preoccupation with health
    3 = Frequent complaints, requests for help, etc.
    4 = Hypochondriacal delusions
(16) LOSS OF WEIGHT: rate either A or B
(A) When rating by history:
    0 = No weight loss
    1 = Probably weight loss associated with present illness
    2 = Definite (according to patient) weight loss
    3 = Not assessed
(B) On weekly ratings by ward psychiatrist, when actual weight changes are measured:
    0 = Less than 1 lb (0.5 kg) weight loss in week
    1 = Greater than 1 lb (0.5 kg) weight loss in week
    2 = Greater than 2 lb (1 kg) weight loss in week
    3 = Not assessed
(17) INSIGHT
    0 = Acknowledges being depressed and ill
    1 = Acknowledges illness but attributes cause to bad food, climate, overwork,
       virus, need for rest, etc.
    2 = Denies being ill at all.

Note: Moderate depression usually indicated by a score of 17 or above.
Source: Hamilton (1960).

website www.psychguides.com/ provides the outline (click on Available Guidelines then Depressive Disorders in Older Patients) and the full guidance can be purchased from this link.

Under the auspices of its Sections of Old Age Psychiatry and Affective Disorder, the World Health Organization has produced a guideline book for late-life depression (Baldwin *et al.* 2002). Google, with permission of the publisher, has sample chapters for the interested reader to view. Go to Google Book Search (http://books.google.com/) and type in Guidelines on Depression in Older People (you may need to register with Google).

A shorter guideline using similar principles to the above was released by the Faculty of Old Age Psychiatry of the UK Royal College of Psychiatrists in the form of a journal article (Baldwin *et al.* 2003). Those with journal access rights (for example some forms of Athens password) can download it.

'Expert review: Pharmacological treatment of depression in older people' is written for *CNS Forum* magazine (2005) by Stephen Curran, a UK old-age

Table 7.8 The Montgomery Äsberg Depression Rating Scale (MADRAS)

(1) Apparent sadness
Reflected in speech, facial expression, and posture. Rate by depth and inability to
brighten up.
> 0 No sadness.
>
> 1
>
> 2 Looks dispirited but does brighten up without difficulty.
>
> 3
>
> 4 Appears sad and unhappy most of the time.
>
> 5
>
> 6 Looks miserable all the time. Extremely despondent.

(2) Reported sadness
Representing reports of depressed mood, regardless of whether it is reflected in
appearance or not. Includes low spirits, despondency or the feeling of being beyond
help and without hope. Rate according to intensity, duration and the extent to
which the mood is reported to be influenced by events.
> 0 Occasional sadness in keeping with the circumstances.
>
> 1
>
> 2 Sad or low but brightens up without difficulty.
>
> 3
>
> 4 Pervasive feelings of sadness or gloominess. The mood is still influenced by
> external circumstances.
>
> 5
>
> 6 Continuous or unvarying sadness, misery or despondency.

(3) Inner tension
Representing feelings of ill-defined discomfort, edginess, inner turmoil, mental
tension mounting to either panic, dread or anguish. Rate according to intensity,
frequency, duration and the extent of reassurance called for.
> 0 Placid. Only fleeting inner tension.
>
> 1
>
> 2 Occasional feelings of edginess and ill-defined discomfort.
>
> 3
>
> 4 Continuous feelings of inner tension or intermittent panic which the patient
> can only master with some difficulty.
>
> 5
>
> 6 Unrelenting dread or anguish. Overwhelming panic.

(4) Reduced sleep
Representing the experience of reduced duration or depth of sleep compared to the
subject's own normal pattern when well.
> 0 Sleeps as usual.
>
> 1
>
> 2 Slight difficulty dropping off to sleep or slightly reduced, light or fitful sleep.
>
> 3
>
> 4 Sleep reduced or broken by at least two hours.

Table 7.8 (*cont.*)

5

6 Less than two or three hours sleep.

(5) Reduced appetite

Representing the feeling of a loss of appetite compared with when well. Rate by loss of desire for food or the need to force oneself to eat.

0 Normal or increased appetite.

1

2 Slightly reduced appetite.

3

4 No appetite. Food is tasteless.

5

6 Needs persuasion to eat at all.

(6) Concentration difficulties

Representing difficulties in collecting one's thoughts mounting to incapacitating lack of concentration. Rate according to intensity, frequency and degree of incapacity produced.

0 No difficulties in concentrating.

1

2 Occasional difficulties in collecting one's thoughts.

3

4 Difficulties in concentrating and sustaining thought which reduces ability to read or hold a conversation.

5

6 Unable to read or converse without great difficulty.

(7) Lassitude

Representing a difficulty getting started or slowness initiating and performing everyday activities.

0 Hardly any difficulty in getting started. No sluggishness.

1

2 Difficulties in starting activities.

3

4 Difficulties in starting simple routine activities which are carried out with effort.

5

6 Complete lassitude. Unable to do anything without help.

(8) Inability to feel

Representing the subjective experience of reduced interest in the surroundings, or activities that normally give pleasure. The ability to react with adequate emotion to circumstances or people is reduced.

0 Normal interest in the surroundings and in other people

1

2 Reduced ability to enjoy usual interests.

3

4 Loss of interest in the surroundings. Loss of feelings for friends and acquaintances.

Table 7.8 (*cont.*)

5

6 The experience of being emotionally paralysed, inability to feel anger, grief or pleasure and a complete or even painful failure to feel for close relatives and friends.

(*9*) *Pessimistic thoughts*

Representing thoughts of guilt, inferiority, self-reproach, sinfulness, remorse and ruin.

0 No pessimistic thoughts

1

2 Fluctuating ideas of failure, self-reproach or self-deprecation.

3

4 Persistent self-accusations, or definite but still rational ideas of guilt or sin. Increasingly pessimistic about the future.

5

6 Delusions of ruin, remorse or unredeemable sin. Self-accusations which are absurd and unshakeable.

(*10*) *Suicidal thoughts*

Representing the feeling that life is not worth living, that a natural death would be welcome, suicidal thoughts, and preparations for suicide. Suicidal attempts should not in themselves influence the rating.

0 Enjoys life or takes it as it comes.

1

2 Weary of life. Only fleeting suicidal thoughts.

3

4 Probably better off dead. Suicidal thoughts are common, and suicide is considered as a possible solution, but without specific plans or intention.

5

6 Explicit plans for suicide when there is an opportunity. Active preparations for suicide.

Note: Moderate depression usually indicated by a score of 20 or greater.
Source: Montgomery and Äsberg (1979). Reprinted with kind permission of the Royal College of Psychiatrists.

psychiatrist. It provides quite detailed information about current antidepressants used to treat depression and is available online: (www.cnsforum.com/magazine/asktheexpert/old_age_depression/).

Consensus Guidelines for Assessment and Management of Depression in the Elderly Faculty of Psychiatry of Old Age, NSW Branch, Royal Australian and New Zealand College of Psychiatrists is a short guide with a number of useful algorithms, including ones on assessment (including suicide risk evaluation) and treatment (www.health.nsw.gov.au/policy/cmh/publications/depression/depression_elderly.pdf; otherwise go to the main New South Wales website and follow links from Centre for Mental Health).

The Canadian Coalition for Seniors' Mental Health (CCSMH) mentioned earlier and in Shulman and Upshur's commentary provides detailed guidelines on three relevant aspects: Assessment and Treatment of Depression; The Assessment and Treatment of Mental Health Issues in Long-Term Care Homes (with a focus on mood and behavioural symptoms); and the Assessment of Suicide Risk and Prevention of Suicide, as discussed above. These are freely available (subject to registering on the website) by following the National Guideline Initiative link from the main website (www.ccsmh.ca/).

The Depression Practice Guideline (2004) of the Ministry of Health of Singapore, developed in association with the Singapore Psychiatric Association, has a short chapter on older patients and includes a basic depression management algorithm (www.moh.gov.sg/cmaweb/attachments/publication/28da14c777BN/ Depression_0.pdf; alternatively go to the main government website and follow links 'statistics, Publications and Resources – Guidelines – Clinical Practice Guidelines 2004').

The British Association of Psychopharmacology (BAP) has a useful guideline on depression although at the time of writing it is being updated (www.bap. org.uk/ and follow the links to Consensus Statements).

In the UK the National Institute of Health and Clinical Excellence (NICE) (www.nice.org.uk/) has issued clinical guidelines on a number of relevant topics. They include unipolar depression (2004), bipolar disorder (2006), electroconvulsive treatment (ECT) (2003) and self-harm (2004).

Best Treatment is a website which produces information from *British Medical Journal*'s Clinical Evidence: www.besttreatments.co.uk/btuk/conditions/1665.html. Using a mouse click the viewer can see the evidence from the perspective of either patient or doctor.

Bipolar disorder

Although bipolar disorder is not a primary focus of this book, depression is one of the major causes of disability in patients with bipolar disorder. The BAP (above) has downloadable guidance as does the National Institute of Health and Clinical Excellence (NICE). The American Psychiatric Association (2002) also has a practice guideline from 2002 which is available to purchase from the APA website with an online update issued in 2005 (www.psych.org/psych_pract/ treatg/pg/Bipolar.watch.pdf). Young *et al.* have written an evidence-based report on bipolar disorder in later life (Young *et al.*, 2004) and there are evidence-based guidelines for treating bipolar disorder (Goodwin 2003).

Patient education material

Relevant literature and online resources

The Geriatric Depression Scale (GDS) can be completed online via the GDS website (www.stanford.edu/~yesavage: follow links to testing page).

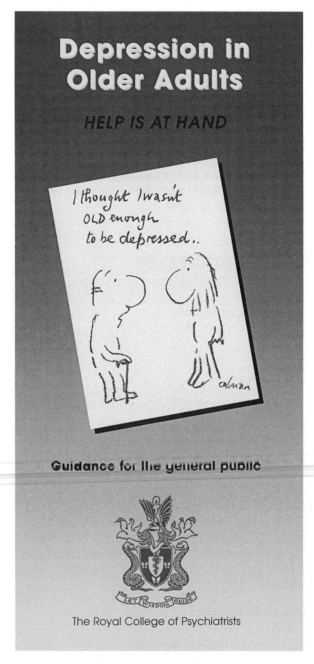

Figure 7.1 'Depression in Older Adults' leaflet reproduced with permission by Royal College of Psychiatrists (c) 2003, artwork (c) S. and C. Calman.

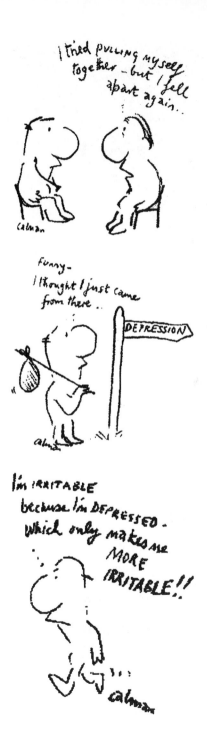

Figure 7.1 (cont)

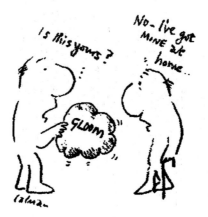

Figure 7.1 (cont)

The American Association for Geriatric Psychiatry has material on depression available through the website of the Geriatric Mental Health Foundation (GMHF): A Guide to Mental Wellness in Older Age: Recognizing and Overcoming Depression (A Depression Recovery Toolkit) and Depression in Late Life: Not a Natural Part of Aging (also available in Spanish) (www.gmhfonline.org/gmhf/consumer/index.html) or go to the GMHF website (www.gmhfonline.org) and follows links to Consumer/Patient information. The GMHF website also contains a number of useful links to other North American organizations.

Also from the United States, as part of the Expert Consensus Group led by George Alexopoulos and colleagues (above), a guide for patients and care givers is available free at www.psychguides.com/ (click on Available Guidelines then Depressive Disorders in Older Patients and finally the Guide)

The Health Minds, Healthy Lives Initiative of the American Psychiatric Association also has generic patient information leaflets (downloadable) for depression and bipolar disorder as part of its 'Let's Talk Facts' series (www.healthyminds.org/) or go to the American Psychiatric Association website and follow links to Public Information.

CANMAT (Canadian Network for Mood and Anxiety Treatments) is a not-for-profit research organization linking health-care professionals from across Canada who have a special interest in mood and anxiety disorders. Its website mainly offers brief patient-oriented information about a range of common mental disorders, including depression in later life (www.canmat.org).

Also from Canada is the Check Up from the Neck Up initiative which has information about self-assessment and overviews of treatment options in depression (www.checkupfromtheneckup.ca/).

The Black Dog Institute is an educational, research, clinical and community-oriented facility based in Australia dedicated to improving understanding, diagnosis and treatment of mood disorders. It produces a number of fact sheets, including one on depression in old age: www.blackdoginstitute.org.au/factsheets/documents/DepressioninOlderPeople.pdf.

In the UK, the Royal College of Psychiatrists produces accessible patient information, again including one on depression in later life (www.rcpsych.ac.uk/pdf/DOA.pdf). In addition to the practice guideline described above, the Singapore Health Ministry also has an online (pdf file) for patients. The file is large and may not download easily but could be useful as it is translated into several locally spoken languages.

Self-help material and groups

The following is a small selection from the UK of the enormous range of resources which are available on the Internet. The list is purely illustrative. Many of the patient information sheets and downloadable documents mentioned above have country-specific information about relevant organizations.

Depression Alliance

212 Spitfire Studios, 63–71 Collier Street, London N1 9BE

Tel: 0845 123 2320 Website: www.depressionalliance.org

This provides information, support and understanding to those who are affected by depression.

Saneline

Tel: 0845 767 8000 Website: www.sane.org.uk

Saneline is a national out-of-hours telephone helpline providing information and support for anyone affected by mental health problems including families and carers.

National Association for Mental Health

MIND, PO Box 277, Manchester M60 3XN

Tel: 0845 766 0163 Website: www.mind.org.uk

Provides a variety of information including generic leaflets on depression, drugs to treat depression and differentiating confusion, depression and dementia. Information is available in: Albanian, Arabic, Bengali, Chinese, Farsi, French, Gujarati, Hindi, Japanese, Punjabi, Somali, Spanish, Turkish, Urdu and Welsh.

The British Association of Behavioural and Cognitive Psychotherapies (BABCP)

Globe Centre, PO Box 9, Accrington BB5 2GD

Tel: 01254 87527 Website: www.babcp.com

The organization maintains a register of qualified practitioners and has a series of pamphlets (available for a small charge) on anxiety, depression, insomnia, understanding CBT and bipolar disorder to mention a few.

Oxford Cognitive Therapy Centre (OCTC)
Based in the Oxford Psychology Department, part of Oxfordshire Mental Healthcare NHS Trust, UK
Website: www.octc.co.uk
The website gives details of how to order a number of educational and self-help booklets with a CBT approach for a range of conditions including depression.
Self-help leaflets based on a CBT approach
Website: www.nnt.nhs.uk/mh/content.asp?PageName=selfhelp
These leaflets are written by members of the Newcastle, North Tyneside and Northumberland Mental Health NHS Trust, UK. This website has useful information and clear leaflets about common mental health issues including depression and bereavement.
Ultrasis
Website: www.ultrasis.com
This organization produces interactive, computer-based CBT programmes for health-care professionals, corporations and consumers, including Beating the Blues which has been endorsed for mild to moderate depression by the National Institute for Health and Clinical Excellence (NICE 2006b).

Self-help manuals

An important part of stepped care (Chapter 2) is the use of self-help which may be facilitated or guided by the health professional. A facilitated self-help intervention with a manual called SHADE, developed for use in adults of working age (Mead *et al.* 2005), has been used by the editors with older people (Chew-Graham *et al.* 2007). The modalities covered include: cognitive restructuring, behavioural activation and relaxation. An example of an Internet-based self-help manual using a similar approach is the Heart of Birmingham Primary Care Trust Self-Help Guide for Depression (www.hobtpct.nhs.uk/your_health/mental_health/docs/Self%20Help%20Guide%20-%20Depression.doc). It is not specific to older people but like the SHADE manual has a large typeface. It covers identifying negative thoughts, challenging and balancing thoughts, activity planning, recording what has been achieved and enjoyed, problem-solving and relaxation.

Not every element of manuals such as these is necessary for every patient. In our experience it is often best to involve a practitioner who can help the patient choose which parts suit them best.

Services for older people with depression

Cole and Yaffe (1996) describe the need to develop pathways of care to improve the care of older people. Table 7.9 lists the major service components

Table 7.9 Major service components to consider in the assessment and management of late-life depression

---

- Medical
  - Primary care
  - General medicine
  - Geriatric medicine
  - General psychiatry (adults of all ages)
  - Old-age (geriatric) psychiatry (age-related services)
- Social care agencies (usually state-aided or funded)
- Voluntary services (usually charitable)
- Religious organizations

---

that should be considered when service development or reconfiguration is under consideration. Although there is variation between countries, the commentators agree that the mainstream *medical* services involved in the assessment and management of late-life depression are primary care, the medical specialties (whether general internal medicine or age-related geriatric medicine) and psychiatry. The psychiatric component may be from generic adult psychiatry services or more specialized age-related services (old age or geriatric psychiatry). Funded *social care* tends to be needs- rather than diagnosis-led. The role of the *voluntary sector* is much more variable and may include advocacy, advice, information and support including practical, emotional and spiritual (especially, but not exclusively, within religious organizations).

The contribution by Lambat (page 77) illustrates how a voluntary organization can address *barriers* to receiving help, in this case in a minority group. Contributors also mention the importance in many cultures of *religious organizations* in providing spiritual and practical support. Resources, however good, can be ineffective if barriers are not identified and addressed. These are discussed in Chapter 1 (Waheed) and by Rait and Lambert in commentaries on Case 4.4; a summary checklist is provided in Table 7.10.

These barriers especially disadvantage poor and minority populations who tend to have more ill-health and are more disabled. In Western societies, African Americans, African Caribbeans, Hispanics, Latinos and Asians are less likely to use mental health services than are Whites (Rait *et al.* 1996, Unützer *et al.* 1999).

In England, Age Concern has a special initiative on black and minority ethnic (BME) elders on its website (www.ageconcern.org.uk/AgeConcern/BME.asp). The UK mental health charity MIND also has information on the mental health of the South Asian community in Britain (www.mind.org.uk/Information/Factsheets/Diversity/MHSACB.htm#organisations).

Table 7.10 Barriers to consider in service delivery

Factors	Possible barriers
Patient-related	Somatization
	Fear of stigmatization
	Negative beliefs about antidepressant medication (for example, addictive)
	False normalization of depression
Practitioner-related	Poor consultation skills
	False normalization of depression
	'Therapeutic nihilism'
	Attribution to societal ills
	Lack of confidence and/or experience in treatments
	Blinkered approach (thinking the problem is either 'physical' or 'mental')
Organizational	Separation of mental health and medical services
	Poor co-ordination of services
	Lack of appropriate services (for example psychological interventions)
	Low reimbursement rates for psychotropic medication
Societal	National legislation regarding age discrimination

Legal framework

Mental capacity

Details about mental capacity and its assessment are beyond the scope of this book and subject to national legislation. However, the need to assess the depressed patient's capacity for decision-making in regard to treatments for depression has been raised by several commentators. In England a new Mental Capacity Act 2005 has set the legal framework. Information is available on the Department of Constitutional Affairs website (www.dca.gov.uk/menincap/legis.htm). A summary of some key points is listed in Table 7.11.

Mental health law

Again, different jurisdictions have their own laws with different histories. For example, Tataru and colleagues mention that mental health law in Romania only came into being in 2002. In England, the Mental Health Act 1983 sets the legislative framework but is under review. Internet guides are available, for example Nigel Turner's popular Hyperguide (www.hyperguide.co.uk/mha/).

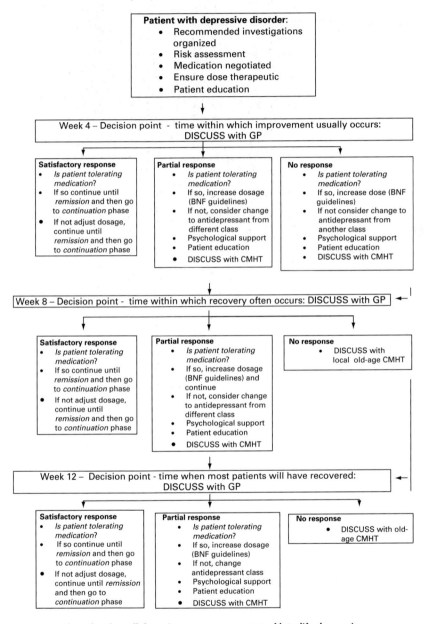

Figure 7.2 Algorithm for collaborative care management of late-life depression.
BNF, British National Formulary; CMHT, community mental health team.

Table 7.11 Principles and guidance about capacity assessments from the Mental Capacity Act 2005 in England

---

Assume a person has capacity unless proved otherwise

Do not treat people as incapable of making a decision unless you have tried all you can to help them

Do not treat someone as incapable of making a decision because their decision may seem unwise

Do things or take decisions for people without capacity in their best interests

Before doing something to someone or making a decision on their behalf, consider whether you could achieve the outcome in a less restrictive way

Key principle is that all decisions must be made in the best interests of the person who lacks capacity, taking into consideration all relevant circumstances

The Act does not define best interests but does give a checklist:

- Must involve the person who lacks capacity
- Have regard for past and present wishes and feelings
- Consult with others who are involved in the care of the person
- Undertake the assessment under circumstances which maximize the person's capabilities
- Document the decision and review it as necessary

Protocols and pathways

To be effective, pathways and protocols should be designed collaboratively by local stakeholders (ideally primary care, specialist services, social care agencies, user groups and the voluntary sector). A protocol and pathway for depression developed collaboratively between primary care and specialist mental health services for older people in Manchester, UK can be found at www.manchesterpct.nhs.uk/.

The stepped care model (Chapter 2) provides a framework for deciding which level of treatment the patient needs. Ideally each step should be supported by a treatment protocol or algorithm for managing the patient. Figure 7.2 provides an example from the editors' locality, and an example from France on page 150.

In summary, practitioners can choose from several validated instruments, available in a variety of languages, to screen for depression and, if they wish, to assess the severity of cases identified on screening. Once available only in printed form, there is now a variety of online literature covering guidelines, self-help literature and sources of support. This steadily accumulating resource looks set to enrich practice with benefit both to patients with late-life depression and those who treat them.

REFERENCES

Abas M., Phillips C., Carter J., *et al.* (1998) Culturally sensitive validation of screening questionnaires for depression in older African-Caribbean people living in South London. *Br. J. Psychiatry* **173**, 249–54.

Adshead F., Day Cody P., Pitt B. (1992) BASDEC: a novel screening instrument for depression in elderly medical inpatient. *Br. Med. J.* **305**, 397.

Alexopoulos G. S., Katz I. R., Reynolds C. F., Carpenter D., Docherty J. P. (2001) *The Expert Consensus Guideline Series: Pharmacotherapy of Depressive Disorders in Older Patients*, Postgrad Med Special Report 2001. Available online at www.psychguides.com/

American Psychiatric Association (1994) *Diagnostic and Statistical Manual*, Version IV. Washington, DC: APA.

American Psychiatric Association (2002) Practice guidelines for the treatment of patients with bipolar disorder. *Am. J. Psychiatry* **159** (Suppl. 4), 1–50.

Baldwin R. C., Chiu E., Katona C., Graham N. (2002) *Guidelines on Depression in Older People: Practising the Evidence.* London: Martin Dunitz.

Baldwin R. C., Anderson D., Black S., *et al.* (2003) Guideline for the management of late-life depression in primary care. *Int. J. Geriatr. Psychiatry* **18**, 829–38.

Beck A. T., Ward C. H., Mendelson M., Mock J. E., Erbaugh J. (1961) An inventory for measuring depression. *Arch. Gen. Psychiatry* **4**, 561–71.

Bird A. S., Macdonald A. J. D., Mann A. H., Philpot M. P. (1987) Preliminary experiences with the SelfCARE(D). *Int. J. Geriatr. Psychiatry* **2**, 31–8.

Bonsignore M., Barkow K., Jessen F., Heun R. (2001) Validity of the five-item WHO Well-Being Index (WHO-5) in an elderly population. *Eur. Arch. Psychiatr. Clin. Neurosci.* **251** (Suppl. 2), II/27–II/31.

Brooke P., Bullock R. (1999) Validation of the 6-Item Cognitive Impairment Test. *Int. J. Geriatr. Psychiatry* **14**, 936–40.

Chew-Graham C. A., Lovell K., Roberts C., *et al.* (2007) A randomized controlled trial to test the feasibility of a collaborative care model for the management of depression in older people. *Br. J. Gen. Practice* **57**, 364–70.

Cole M. G., Yaffe M. J. (1996) Pathway to psychiatric care of the elderly with depression. *Int. J. Geriatr. Psychiatry* **11**, 157–61.

Folstein M. F., Folstein S. E., McHugh P. R. (1975) 'Mini-Mental State': a practical method for grading the cognitive state of patients for the clinician. *J. Psychiatr. Res.* **12**, 185–98.

Goodwin G. M., for the Consensus Group of the British Association for Psychopharmacology (2003) Evidence-based guidelines for treating bipolar disorder: recommendations from the British Association for Psychopharmacology. *J. Psychopharmacol.* **17**, 149–73.

Hamilton M. (1960) A rating scale for depression. *J. Neurol. Neurosurg. Psychiatry* **23**, 56–62.

Katzman R., Brown T., Fuld P., *et al.* (1983) Validation of a short Orientation–Memory–Concentration Test of cognitive impairment. *Am. J. Psychiatry* **140**, 734–9.

Kroenke K., Spitzer R. L., Williams J. B. (2001) The PHQ-9: validity of a brief depression severity measure. *J. Gen. Intern. Med.* **16**, 606–13.

Krishnan K. R. R., Delong M., Kraemer H., *et al.* (2002) Comorbidity of depression with other medical diseases in the elderly. *Biol. Psychiatry* **52**, 559–88.

Marin R. S., Biedrzycki R. C., Firinciogullari S. (1991) Reliability and validity of the Apathy Evaluation Scale. *Psychiatr. Res.* **38**, 143–62.

Mead N., Macdonald W., Bower P., *et al.* (2005) The clinical effectiveness of guided self-help versus waiting-list control in the management of anxiety and depression: a randomized controlled trial. *Psychol. Med.* **35**, 1633–43.

Montgomery S. A., Äsberg M. (1979) A new depression scale designed to be sensitive to change. *Br. J. Psychiatry* **134**, 382–9.

NICE (2003) *The Clinical Effectiveness and Cost Effectiveness of Electroconvulsive Therapy (ECT) for Depressive Illness, Schizophrenia, Catatonia and Mania*, Health Technology Assessment No. 59. London: National Institute for Health and Clinical Excellence.

NICE (2004a) *Self-Harm: The Short-Term Physical and Psychological Management and Secondary Prevention of Self-Harm in Primary and Secondary Care*, Clinical Guideline No. 16. London: National Institute for Health and Clinical Excellence.

NICE (2004b) *Depression: Management of Depression in Primary and Secondary Care*, Clinical Guideline No. 23. London: National Institute for Health and Clinical Excellence.

NICE (2006a) *Depression and Anxiety: Computerized Cognitive Behavioural Therapy (CCBT)*, Health Technology Assessment No. 97. London: National Institute for Health and Clinical Excellence.

NICE (2006b) *Bipolar Disorder: The Management of Bipolar Disorder in Adults, Children and Adolescents, in Primary and Secondary care*, Clinical Guideline No. 38. London: National Institute for Health and Clinical Excellence.

Radloff L. S. (1977) The CES-D scale: a self-report depression scale for research in the general population. *Appl. Psychol. Measurement* **1**, 385–401.

Rait G., Burns A., Chew C. A. (1996) Old age, ethnicity and mental illness: a triple whammy. *Br. Med. J.* **313**, 1347–8.

Rait G., Burns A., Baldwin R., *et al.* (1999) Screening for depression in older African-Caribbeans. *Fam. Practice* **16**, 591–5.

Shulman K. I. (2000) Clock-drawing: is it the ideal cognitive screening test? *Int. J. Geriatr. Psychiatry* **15**, 548–61.

Unützer J., Katon W., Sullivan M., Miranda J. (1999) Treating depressed older adults in primary care: narrowing the gap between efficacy and effectiveness. *Millbank Q.* **77**, 225–56.

Young R. C., Gyulai L., Mulsant B. H., *et al.* (2004) Pharmacotherapy of bipolar disorder in old age. *Am. J. Geriatr. Psychiatry* **12**, 342–57.

Watson L. C., Pigmore M. P. (2003) Screening accuracy for late-life depression in primary care: a systematic review. *J. Fam. Practice* **52**, 956–64.

Williams E. I., Wallace P. (1993) *Health Checks for People Aged 75 and Over*, Occasional Paper No. 59, British Journal of Geriatric Practice.

FURTHER READING

Burroughs H., Morley M., Lovell K., *et al.* (2006) 'Justifiable depression': how health professionals and patients view late-life depression; a qualitative study. *Fam. Practice* **23**, 369–77.

Iliffe S., Lenihan P., Orrell M., *et al.* and the SPICE Research Team (2004) The development of a short instrument to identify common unmet needs in older people in general practice. *Br. J. Gen. Practice* **54**, 914–18.

Kato T. (2005) [Suicide prevention for patients with depressive disorder in Japan.] *Seishin Shinkeigaku Zasshi* **107**, 1069–77.

Royal College of Physicians and British Geriatric Society (1992) *Standardized Assessment Scales for Elderly People*, Report of the Joint Workshops of the Research Unit of the Royal College of Physicians and the British Geriatric Society. London: Royal College of Physicians.

Spitzer R., Kroenke K., Williams J. (1999) Validation and utility of a self-report version of PRIME-MD: the PHQ Primary Care Study. *J. Am. Med. Assoc.* **282**, 1737–44.

Unützer J., Katon W., Callahan C. M., *et al.* (2002) Collaborative care management of late life depression in the primary care setting. *J. Am. Med. Assoc.* **288**, 2836–45.

World Health Organization (1993) *The ICD-10 Classification of Mental and Behavioural Disorders: Research Criteria*. Geneva: WHO.

Appendix: International commentaries

The editors summarized the contributions written by colleagues in different parts of the world (Chapter 6) to illustrate the similarities, and occasional differences, in the management of depression in older people described in all the contributions. This appendix allows the reader to read the individual contributions.

Australia

Professor David Ames, Professor of Psychiatry of Old Age, University of Melbourne, and Dr Eleanor Flynn, Senior Lecturer in Medical Education, University of Melbourne

Assessment

This 82-year-old woman is chronically disabled by pain and breathlessness and appears to have become socially disengaged. She has several symptoms of depression, including persistent low mood, loss of energy (which sounds to be out of proportion to her medical state), early morning waking, loss of interest in previously enjoyed activities, and persistent feelings that life is not worth living. The vignette does not provide information about her appetite and weight, concentration, any psychomotor changes, guilt feelings or confidence levels, but even so it is clear that, provided the symptoms have been present for two weeks (and this seems highly likely), she meets both DSM-IV diagnostic criteria for a major depressive episode and ICD-10 criteria for a depressive episode.

Australian health-care system

Within the Australian health-care system, in which specialists are accessible only after referral from a general practitioner (GP), this woman would

Integrated Management of Depression in the Elderly, ed. C. Chew-Graham, R. Baldwin and A. Burns. Published by Cambridge University Press. © Cambridge University Press 2008.

normally be managed by her GP who in all likelihood will already be engaged in the management of her troublesome osteoarthritis and chronic obstructive pulmonary disease (COPD). She might well attend a respiratory outpatient clinic or rheumatology clinic in a public hospital, or (less likely as fewer than one-third of the elderly have private health insurance) be seeing a private medical specialist with expertise in one or both of these two areas. Referral to a public old-age psychiatry team would be unlikely (especially outside of the state of Victoria, or if she lived outside a capital city) unless she had not improved on a GP-prescribed antidepressant. The first author's old-age psychiatry service, covering 45 000 individuals aged above 65, receives approximately 700 new referrals for assessment each year. Yet taking a very conservative estimate of 1% of the elderly being affected by a major depressive disorder (Ames 2001), one would expect there to be at least 450 old people with major depression within that catchment area at any given time, with a significant turnover of incident and recovering cases (even though many may be chronic). As the bulk of referrals received are for people with dementia and disturbed behaviour, and a large proportion of the remaining referrals are for people with schizophrenia and related disorders, clearly the majority of elderly individuals with major depression are not being referred, despite the fact that this catchment has one of the most active, engaged community aged psychiatry services in the country.

It is unlikely that Miss LC would see a geriatrician unless she were referred to an old-age care assessment service (LoGiudice *et al.* 2005) in order to be considered for residential accommodation designed to meet a higher level of need.

Assessment by most GPs would involve taking a history and performing a mental state examination, with a strong focus on assessing any suicide risk and expressed intention of deliberate self-harm, though such assessment would typically be brief, as the current system of GP remuneration rewards multiple short consultations much more generously than a small number of long ones. Encouragingly, recent funding changes now reward GPs quite well for attendance at multidisciplinary case meetings for patients over the age of 75 years.

Undergraduate training in psychiatry has been of reasonably high quality in most Australian medical schools since the early 1960s, and in the past 15 years GPs have been subject to a large range of educational initiatives with regard to depression, many of which were funded by the pharmaceutical industry. One such initiative among GPs in attendance to a Sydney residential home complex showed some evidence of modest, sustained benefit in the reduction of rates of depression among 1036 older residents (Llewellyn-Jones *et al.* 1999).

Management

In managing this patient we would take account of her frailty and apparent social isolation and would consider her other medications, especially the possibility that they might interact with any antidepressant we would wish to prescribe. We would also be concerned to make an in-depth inquiry about any suicidal ideation and to assess carefully her suicide risk at a very early stage of the assessment.

First-line treatment at GP level for this lady would be likely to involve prescription of an antidepressant. The most commonly prescribed antidepressant in Australia is sertraline and a majority of GPs would initiate this drug at dose of 25 mg mane (each morning) before increasing the dose to 50 mg mane after one or two weeks.

In common with many other countries, Australia has seen a marked increase in the rate of antidepressant prescribing over the past 15 years, since the introduction of the selective serotonin reuptake inhibitors (SSRIs) and other novel classes of antidepressant drugs. Access to cognitive behavioural therapy (CBT) is very limited by the small number of practitioners available and willing to work with older people (our local old-age psychiatry service does not at present employ a clinical psychologist with expertise in CBT), but new reimbursement regulations made in the 2006 Australian Federal Government budget now permit the direct referral by GPs of patients direct to private clinical psychologists for a limited number of treatment sessions, the cost of which will be now be covered by the national universal health insurance scheme 'Medicare'. It is likely that there will be steady growth in the use of CBT to treat depressions such as Miss LC's in future years.

Guidelines

A number of sets of guidelines for the treatment of depression (most not focussed exclusively upon the elderly) have been developed by the Royal Australian College of GPs, the Royal Australian and New Zealand College of Psychiatrists and the government-funded public health depression initiative Beyond Blue (www.beyondblue.org.au), and these can be consulted online, but it is fair to say that their utilization would be 'a custom more honoured in the breach than in the observance'.

Roles of primary and secondary care

The roles of the two authors in the management of this patient would differ. As a GP, EF would be responsible for the total medical care of the patient, liaison with any specialist or support services involved, and would prescribe medications. As a specialist in psychiatry of old age DA would expect to see the patient for an opinion and would advise the GP on management. He also would undertake liaison with a nursing or allied health staff member of the aged psychiatry community team, and would review the patient if she did not improve with treatment. He could offer inpatient assessment and treatment in a publicly funded 20-bed acute old-age psychiatry unit should her depression deteriorate, or if the risk of suicide was very high.

The Australian health-care system does aim to provide equitable access to health care for all Australians though the Medicare system. Resource availability restricts this aim. Access to private specialists is limited by geography (there are very few psychiatrists in rural areas and they are in short supply in the less affluent areas of the major cities), financial resources, and a tendency for private psychiatrists to want to see young and middle-aged adults rather than elderly people. Victoria State has well-established publicly funded specialist aged psychiatry services which are free at the point of delivery, but other states do not all have comparable services. But probably the biggest barrier to effective treatment remains recognition by patients, families and health workers.

REFERENCES

Ames D. (2001) Depression and the elderly. In *Depression: Social and Economic Timebomb*, eds. A. Dawson and A. Tylee. London: BMJ Books, pp. 49–54.

Llewellyn-Jones R., Baike K., Smithers H., Cohen J., Snowdon J. (1999) Multifaceted shared care intervention for late-life depression in residential care: randomized controlled trial. *Br. Med. J.* **319**, 676–82.

LoGiudice D., Flynn E., Ames D. (2005) Services to people with dementia: a worldwide view – Australia. In *Dementia*, eds. A. Burns, J. O'Brien and D. Ames. London: Hodder Arnold, pp. 256–60.

Bulgaria

Professor Maria Alekxandrova, Associate Professor of Psychiatry, Medical University, Pleven, and Dr Kaloyan Stoychev, Consultant Psychiatrist, University Hospital, Pleven

Diagnosis

Probably due to atypical presentations in later life coupled with much physical co-morbidity, physicians often under-diagnose depression in our health system, where most patients are first seen by their GP. Although there are good assessment tools like the Geriatric Depression Scale and the Hamilton Depression Rating Scale they are rarely used in primary care.

Assessment

For Miss LC, the main factors I would take into account are: her isolation and solitary living, despite being in a sheltered facility, probably due to physical slowing and tiredness; her poor health from osteoarthritis and chronic obstructive pulmonary disease (COPD) which limits participation in social activities; her poor sleep quality; and the risk of suicide (she has thought that life is not worth living).

Management

The main non-pharmacological approaches to be pursued are: attending to her social care needs (especially loneliness and social isolation), whilst at the same time using this as an opportunity for others to make sure she is safe; educating care-givers about depression; treating her concurrent physical health problems via primary care and relevant specialist referral; reducing as much as possible the effects of handicap caused by these conditions (by proper analgesia, pharmacological treatment of the pulmonary disease, etc.); organizing appropriate social care agencies which can help; prompt hospitalization if adequate support and observation can not be achieved in the patient's residence.

Selective serotonin reuptake inhibitors (SSRIs) are drugs of choice in this country because of their tolerability and side effect profile. In the first several weeks of the treatment course, an adjuvant therapy with small dose of benzodiazepine (clonazepam 0.5 mg daily, preferably in the evening) may be given followed by gradual withdrawal. If there is no improvement in four to six weeks, dose increase would be offered or another antidepressant from another class should be tried. Possible second-line options are venlafaxine, mirtazapine, buspiron and tricyclic antidepressants. Although psychological therapies are recommended they are seldom available in this country structured psychotherapy is offered only for psychiatric inpatients at university psychiatric departments, state psychiatric hospitals and regional mental health centres but there are only five university psychiatric clinics, nine psychiatric hospitals (most of which are situated outside the major cities) and 13 regional mental health centres (from 28 main administrative districts).

Supportive psychotherapy is the main method of psychological intervention: the therapist role includes showing interest, concern, empathy, encouragement and acceptance but also tackling specific problems and helping point the patient to relevant services. Typically this is offered weekly although in primary care GPs may use their opportunistic consultations, for example to check blood pressure, to achieve some of these therapeutic aims. Cognitive therapy, based on the well-known negative triad concerning oneself, negative interpretations of experience and a negative view of the future, is practised but at a pace that is usually slower than with younger adults, often with a therapeutic alliance forged through the younger therapist acknowledging the patient's sense of seniority not only in years. The therapeutic role may be more active to help the patient focus more on the here and now than on reminiscence.

Referral to secondary care

Miss LC would only be referred to a psychiatrist if her depression is of at least moderate severity and there has been no benefit from antidepressant treatment within four to six weeks or if psychological support or psychotherapy has not worked. Regular contact with primary care is kept, often over the telephone, and important discussions occur around if and when admission to hospital becomes necessary, what kind of drug to augment the therapy, and how long after recovery should it continue. In cases where extreme loneliness has precipitated the depressive episode, the psychiatrist and patient's GP will work together to find appropriate accommodation in an assisted-living facility (nursing home, etc.). Medical specialists may be involved to address co-morbidity and medication interactions. Lastly, the psychiatrist is also responsible for education of the patient and care-givers about depression and its management.

The barriers to effective treatment are, as discussed, the low sensitivity of GPs to depression in later life and poor communication between them and other medical specialists. There is also a lack of adequately trained staff (nurses and other health-care professionals) in nursing homes and other similar facilities and a shortage of case managers, such as practice nurses, with the skills to co-ordinate care in complex cases such as that of Miss LC.

Canada

Professor Kenneth Shulman, Professor of Geriatric Psychiatry, University of Toronto, and Professor Ross Upshur, Professor of Primary Care, University of Toronto

Co-morbid depression

This 82-year-old lady with significant chronic medical conditions including severe osteoarthritis and chronic obstructive pulmonary disease (COPD) has become symptomatic with shortness of breath and pain affecting her mood and level of functioning. She is quite typical of the growing number of community-dwelling seniors with complex chronic diseases. In addition to her chronic medical illnesses, her history certainly suggests that she may have a co-morbid major depression. Complicating the situation is relative social isolation.

Canadian health-care system

The point of first contact for such an individual in the Canadian health-care system would most likely be a primary care physician (PCP) or a community-based caseworker if she had already been identified by a service in the past. First, the PCP would optimize the medical management of her COPD and osteoarthritis which of itself may have some benefit for her depressive symptoms, including breathlessness, pain and sleep disturbance. Including physical therapy and pulmonary rehabilitation to her regimen may provide the stimulus necessary to get her to go out and hence reduce her social isolation. The primary care physician would also recognize the interaction between somatic illness and depression, would assess depressive symptoms and likely initiate therapy (see below) with close follow-up. Particular focus would be placed on assessing her safety and capacity to manage her affairs including an assessment of her risk of harming herself. A follow up visit would likely be scheduled for two to three weeks hence.

A variety of community resources can be mobilized to maintain contact with the patient and assess progress including outreach services, which in Canada could emanate from the geriatric medical service, the psychogeriatric service or indeed from primary care. A number of health-care professionals including PCPs, nurses, social workers and psychiatrists associated with agencies coordinated by our Community Care Access Centres (CCAC) could be mobilized (www.health.gov.on.ca/english/public/contact/ccac/ccac_mn.html). These individuals or services could address the question of diagnosis of major depression as well as its management and monitor the response of her other chronic illnesses to therapy. A recommendation of admission to a day program may result. Access to a psychiatrist to assess such an individual is available in most major centres in Canada but the proportion of those with depression, at any age, referred to a psychiatrist from a PCP is small.

Guidelines for assessment and management of depression in Canada

At the national level, the Canadian Network for Mood and Anxiety Treatments (CANMAT) has a well-organized approach to the management of patients with depressive and bipolar disorders (Kennedy *et al.* 2001) (see also Chapter 7). These are available for individuals and professionals alike. CANMAT also provides help and resources specifically focussed on older adults including explanations of contributing aetiological factors, risk factors (including for suicide) and a self-assessment guide using the Geriatric Depression Scale (GDS). CANMAT also focusses on the relationship between depression and a number of medical and neurological problems including hypothyroidism, Alzheimer's disease, Parkinson's disease, congestive heart failure and infectious diseases.

An important new resource is a website entitled 'Check Up from the Neck Up' (www.checkupfromtheneckup.ca). This website is a collaborative project of the Mood Disorders Association of Ontario and a number of other organizations including Sunnybrook Health Sciences Centre, University of Toronto where the Chief of Psychiatry, Dr Anthony Levitt, is an important resource for the website. This website provides self-assessment guidelines as well as a summary of available treatments including pharmacological and psychological approaches to the management of depression.

In May 2006, the Canadian Coalition for Seniors' Mental Health (CCSMH) produced a comprehensive document entitled *National Guidelines for Seniors' Mental Health*. This coalition was established in 2002 following a conference hosted by the Canadian Academy of Geriatric Psychiatry (CAGP). They established a guideline development group specifically for depression in older adults led by Dr Marie-France Tourigny Rivard of the University of Ottawa and Dr Diane Buchanan from the School of Nursing at Queen's University, Kingston, Ontario. These guidelines provide recommendations regarding screening and assessment for depression in older adults where specific risk factors are identified. Referring back to the case example, these factors include social isolation, chronic disabling illness, recent major physical illness (within three months), persistent sleep difficulties and significant somatic concerns. Clearly, Miss LC would be identified as at significant risk for a major depression based on these. The guidelines suggest that following a positive screen for depression, a bio-psychosocial assessment should be conducted to include a formal review of diagnostic criteria which in North American means the *Diagnostic and Statistical Manual* of the American Psychiatric Association (DSM-IV) or the World Health Organization's ICD-10 diagnostic manual. Also included are an estimate of the severity of depressive symptomatology, a specific risk assessment for suicide, a functional assessment, a review of personal and family history of mood disorder, a review of medication and substance abuse, and a review of current stressors and life situation, supports available and personal strengths. In addition to the mental status examination, a formal cognitive screen is recommended, either the Mini-Mental State Examination (MMSE) or the clock-drawing test.

There are varying levels of collaboration between PCPs and specialist psychiatric services. Most care for depression is provided by the PCP with referral for refractory cases or concern for more complex psychopathology such as mixed cognitive impairment and mood disorder or lack of clarity with respect to the diagnosis. In Canada, a model of shared care is popular, in which psychiatrists and PCPs work in a collaborative fashion, although the more traditional consultation model is still practised.

Treatment approaches

Evidence suggests that patients with concurrent medical illness respond at least as well as those without significant co-morbid conditions and Canadian guidelines therefore recommend following the same approach as in a general adult population. They also agree that it is important to optimize treatment of concurrent medical disorders (as suggested in this case). The guidelines recommend that the newer antidepressant agents with lower anticholinergic properties should be first-line treatments as they are less likely to cause postural hypotension or cardiac conduction problems. The selective serotonin reuptake inhibitors (SSRIs) as well as venlafaxine, bupropion and mirtazepine are most commonly recommended for those with co-morbid medical illnesses but with caution regarding drug interactions in those with concurrent medical illnesses.

Over-diagnosis

Current evidence in Canada suggests that clinicians, including PCPs, are attuned to the possibility of a major depressive illness in older adults to a much greater extent than used to be the case. If anything, there may be a tendency to over-diagnose depression especially when cognitive impairment is beginning. So there is a need for careful cognitive assessment as well as assessment of depression in such individuals. Overcoming social isolation, as described in this case, remains one of the greatest barriers to the ongoing treatment of depressed patients in our health-care system as community outreach is not as well developed as it should be in most medical and psychiatric services.

REFERENCES

Kennedy S. H., Lam R. W. and the CANMAT Depression Working Group (2001) Clinical guidelines for the treatment of depressive disorders. *Can. J. Psychiatry* **46** (Suppl. 1), 1S–92S.

Canadian Coalition for Seniors' Mental Health (2006) *National Guidelines for Seniors' Mental Health. The Assessment and Treatment of Depression.* Available online at www.ccsmh.ca

Denmark

Dr Kirsten Abelskov, Old-Age Psychiatrist, Aarhus University Hospital, and Dr Kaj Sparle Christensen, General Practitioner, Institut for Almen Medicin, University of Aarhus

The Danish health-care system

In Denmark 98% of people are registered with a general practitioner (GP) and health care is accessed primarily through this route as almost all specialized treatment, including hospital admission, requires GP referral. The only exception is for emergency cases. The Danish health-care system is almost entirely tax financed and most medical care is free. Prescribed medication though is not free as patients have to pay themselves and are reimbursed to 75% of the price of the cheapest generic drug.

Presentation of depression

Depression in older people often presents with physical complaints and impaired social functioning, rather than a direct complaint of low mood.

In the presented case most likely a relative or a home carer would contact the GP by phone and request a home visit. The GP would assess both physical and mental health aspects which is especially important in this case as the patient has co-morbidity which needs careful assessment and optimum management.

Most GPs use ICD-10 criteria for diagnosis and Danish GPs are expected to use the ICD-10 Primary Health Care version (World Health Organization) for the diagnosis of depression. Some use the Geriatric Depression Scale (GDS) for diagnosis and monitoring. The Hamilton Depression Scale may be occasionally used. The use of valid psychometric instruments is financially supported and encouraged in Danish primary care.

Assessment

A full history both of physical problems and mood is needed. The GP particularly needs to explore factors such as loneliness and social support, drugs taken and alcohol use. The patient should be asked what she thinks is wrong. A focussed physical examination is vital to detect significant worsening of known physical health conditions or the development of new physical problems (for example heart failure or weight loss due to malignancy). Blood tests such as full blood count, biochemical profile and thyroid function tests should be undertaken unless the GP has access to very recent results. The GP may also ask a practice nurse to carry out urine tests and an electrocardiogram (ECG), if indicated by the history or physical examination.

If depression is diagnosed, the GP will discuss this with the patient, explain the possible management strategies and explore patient choices in treatment.

Non-drug treatment

Social activities should be encouraged. For example using a wheelchair to increase mobility and facilitate going to a communal room or a church group. Referral of the patient for a psychological intervention can be considered but in reality availability of such services is limited.

First-line drug treatment

If the patient accepts drug treatment, an selective serotonin reuptake inhibitor (SSRI), most often citalopram or sertraline is prescribed. A dual action drug such as venlafaxine, mirtazapine or duloxetine could be prescribed if the GP feels that the depression is moderate to severe, or the patient has failed to respond to an SSRI in the past. Because of side effects, drug interactions and dangers of overdose, tricyclic antidepressants should be avoided.

If the symptoms are not reduced effectively, combination therapy should be considered, although this would be started by a secondary care colleague. Augmentation therapy with lithium is always initiated by the specialist service but the required monitoring can be carried out in primary care.

Guidelines

There are no guidelines for the management of depression in Denmark at present. National guidelines for recognition and treatment of depression are in progress.

Collaboration

If the patient does not improve within three to six weeks or their symptoms are becoming worse, the GP can then contact the 'psychogeriatric hot-line' which is centralized in the city of Risskov. The hot-line is manned by specialists in old-age psychiatry. The advice is in the first instance likely to include a change to the medication or a suggestion to supplement treatment with cognitive therapy. However, the advice might be a referral to the local psychogeriatric hospital, either as outpatient or as inpatient.

Outpatients

Outpatients (office visits) are usually assessed within 1–21 days by a nurse or, if it is a first visit, by a psychiatrist. Outpatients are treated and followed up by a specialized nurse. Patients who have had suicidal attempts will be seen in the outpatient service shortly after discharge from the hospital. Severely depressed patients are seen every week, later every month. Patients with mild depression are seen less frequently and discharged sooner.

Inpatients

Only patients who have not responded to the above treatment strategies or are suicidal are treated as inpatients. Patients are treated medically, managing their physical problems, often with physiotherapy (which is central in this case) and the addition of occupational therapy as well as antidepressant treatment and group psychotherapy.

About 25% of the depressed inpatients are treated with electroconvulsive therapy (ECT). ECT is used if the patient does not respond to intensive drug treatment or if the situation is life-threatening, as when patients are not drinking and eating sufficiently or have made a serious suicidal attempt and are considered at risk of another one.

Information for patients

Depressed patients who are admitted to secondary care are given a leaflet about depression, risk factors, symptoms and treatments. Those treated as inpatients also receive an information leaflet a few days before discharge.

The relatives of depressed patients are given two leaflets, one about how to talk and deal with a depressed relative. A very frequent mistake from relatives is to ask the patient to deal with multiple tasks all at once. The depressed patient may not be able to finish any of the tasks when faced with this and their confidence is further dented. The leaflet advises relatives to give information in bite-size simple chunks. The second leaflet describes symptoms, treatments and myths about depression.

When patients are discharged from the hospital those closely involved with their ongoing recovery are informed and prepared: home nurses (e.g. administration of medication), day care centres (e.g. planned activities), GPs (discharge summary letter) and private physiotherapists (follow-up treatment).

Barriers to effective treatment

Patient barriers include lack of recognition of depression as a problem which can result in not presenting to the GP, not accepting depression as a problem or not complying with prescribed medication. In addition, medication is expensive and has side effects, so patients may make decisions to stop taking their prescribed drugs based on financial considerations.

There are professional or system factors including non-recognition of depression among older people by primary care professionals. In addition, the home care system may prematurely stop providing care to patients if the patient declines such input, or if their mood seems to be improving, even though they continue to need the service.

France

Professor Philippe H. Robert, Professor of Psychiatry, and Dr Michel Benoit, Psychiatrist, Centre Mémoire de Ressources et de Recherche, Nice, Dr Florence Cabane, General Practitioner, Nice, and Dr Geneviève Ruault, Geriatrician, Nice

Pathways of care

The authors represent the disciplines of general medicine, geriatrics and neuropsychiatry which typically may be involved in France in the diagnosis and treatment areas of depression in the older people.

In France Miss LC would most likely consult a general practitioner (GP) and a psychiatrist would only be involved as a second step to confirm the diagnosis and/or the treatment. In France access to the GP is not restricted. To access a specialist there are two options: via the GP or direct access to the specialist but without full reimbursement by the state welfare system. In the future though there will probably be more structured access to specialists. However, the advantage of this dual system is more flexibility which may suit older people who may not be ready to accept a new and more rigid model.

Presentation

Presentations like that of Miss LC are common in France. The major concerns for the GP are: to address co-morbid physical diagnoses and psychiatric diagnoses such as early dementia and to assess psychosocial aspects before starting any pharmacological treatment.

There is not a 'French' presentation of depression, but there are characteristic features in older patients which may alter the classical presentation. These include: the common occurrence of co-morbid somatic diseases; the frequency of somatic preoccupation (as in the case study); the association with cognitive disturbances and memory complaints; the presence of anxiety; feelings of loss of control over the social environment; and the presence of apathy and diminished motivation.

Diagnosis

In March 2006, the Direction Générale de la Santé (DGS) initiated a programme to improve the diagnosis and the treatment of depression. Suggested instruments include the four-item Geriatric Depression Scale (GDS) (Do you feel sad? Do you feel that your life is empty? Do you feel happy most of the time? Do you feel that your situation is hopeless?) and an Apathy Inventory (covering emotional blunting, lack of initiative and lack of interest). In addition an overall assessment must be done including: past medical history; assessment of cognition function using Mini-Mental State Examination (MMSE) or other brief cognitive test; clinical examination and if needed biological and brain-imaging examination (only in the context of a memory clinic or a specialist examination); and a specific assessment of the suicidal risk, from suicidal ideation (episodic or permanent) to the planning of a suicidal act. As in some other countries, GPs do not readily wish to use sophisticated tools which are time-consuming and costly.

Diagnosis and management

The successive steps of diagnosis and management for outpatient are summarized in Figure A.1.

Taking account of co-morbidity, Miss LC is most likely to be treated with a selective serotonin reuptake inhibitor (SSRI), dual-acting antidepressant, tianeptine or moclobemide. If apathy is present, treatment with dual antidepressant or moclobemide may be considered. When prescribing antidepressants other psychotropic drugs such as anxiolytics should be avoided. The explanation given to the patients should encompass the potential benefits of the treatment, not only for depressive symptoms but also for the cognitive and somatic domains. In addition information should also be given about the potential side effects that might be expected. Given the misuse and underuse of antidepressants it is important to underline that Miss LC should continue on the same dosage of antidepressant which led to improvement for at least six months after recovery.

In addition, the following are important: care management information, education about depression to the patient and any carers (if the patient agrees), cognitive behavioural therapy, occupational and social interventions especially to counter social isolation.

Barriers to effective management

The main barrier to effective treatment of the depressed patient is, in France, the non-recognition of the depression or the view that depression is considered as something 'normal' among older people. This is not to underestimate the fact that depressive feelings frequently follow a life event but rather that practitioners find it difficult to differentiate normal sadness from depression as a disorder. This is a training issue and currently there is insufficient time devoted to it. Secondly, we conclude by emphasizing the use of specific tools to assess depression as advocated by the French Ministry of Health.

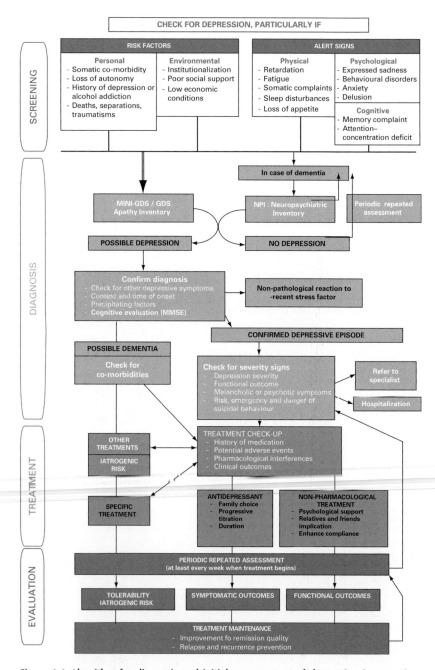

Figure A.1 Algorithm for diagnosis and initial management of depression in outpatient clinics in France.

Hong Kong

Professor Helen F. K. Chiu, Professor of Psychiatry, The Chinese University of Hong Kong, and Professor D. K. T. Li, Family Physician, Past President, Hong Kong College of Family Physicians

Health-care system in Hong Kong

The model of service delivery of old-age psychiatry in Hong Kong is adapted from that of the UK as many old-age psychiatrists were trained there (Chiu *et al.* 1996). A community-oriented multidisciplinary approach is adopted, with close liaison with governmental organizations and geriatric services. In addition to outpatient and inpatient services, there is an outreach programme providing psychiatric services to residents of old-age homes and nursing homes. At present, there are seven psychogeriatric teams funded by the government covering the whole of Hong Kong. However, there are constraints on these services in terms of personnel and funding.

In Hong Kong, the framework of service provision in primary care is different from that in the UK. A sizeable portion of primary medical care providers in Hong Kong are general practitioners (GP) in private practice, many of whom have not yet undergone vocational training in family medicine. Other primary care providers in Hong Kong comprise two groups: (1) doctors who have completed training, and are certified to provide care, in family medicine; (2) non-primary care doctors providing primary care services in private practice. Among the latter are specialists like physicians, obstetricians, gynaecologists, paediatricians, etc., who may sometimes provide limited primary care services. The concept of a 'family doctor' in Hong Kong is only emerging relatively recently and many people still tend to shop around for doctors.

The specialty of family medicine has developed over the last 20 years. This has led to structured vocational training with a number of the family physicians having the opportunity to undergo some training in psychiatry, with several diploma and certificate courses on mental health for primary care doctors. They then become more able to treat patients with mild depression as well as other mood disorders. Recently, the Hong Kong College of Family Physicians has also established a mental health interest group with a forum to provide psychiatric training for primary care doctors.

Presentation

The clinical picture of Miss LC, with her somatic concern, is a common presentation of a depressive illness in Hong Kong. Feelings of sadness and suicidal ideas are seldom articulated spontaneously but the older persons may admit to them if probed sensitively by health-care professionals. Another common feature is the thought of being a burden to the family, which may reflect Chinese culture with its strong family ties. Many local elderly are reluctant to seek help for mental health problems because of the stigma of mental illness and may see it as 'shameful'. They often misconceive it as a sign of morally weakness or 'bad genes' in the family. There is a taboo to seeking help outside the family circle for 'shameful illness and matters' in the Chinese culture. In addition, studies in Asia have also shown that consistent with the high rates of somatization, many older persons who attempt suicide when depressed visit primary care doctors beforehand. Primary care doctors are therefore in a good position to be gate-keepers in the detection of depression and suicidal risk in the older persons (Chiu *et al.* 2003).

Depression is usually recognized by professionals who have received appropriate training in mental health but among the general public there is poor awareness and less vigilance when compared to physical disorder. A common misconception is that feeling depressed is normal for the older persons.

Models of management

Miss LC may already be receiving treatment from her primary care doctor for her chronic obstructive pulmonary disease (COPD) and osteoarthritis. Mild depression may be managed solely by the primary care doctor but more severe depression may lead to referral to a psychiatrist. If the latter, then a referral to a multidisciplinary psychogeriatric team will follow. The old-age psychiatrist serves as the team leader and co-ordinator of treatment plans, with members of the team delivering health and social care interventions. Primary care doctors or GPs in private practice usually work solo in Hong Kong. Shared care or collaborative care models involving psychiatrists and primary care doctors in the management of psychiatric illness are still uncommon. In Hong Kong there is a patient culture which expects quick fixes and the practice of 'doctor shopping' and lack of appreciation of continuous, comprehensive holistic care also make collaborative care difficult to implement successfully.

Assessment

At first assessment a history will be taken covering presenting symptoms, past health, personal and family history, current medications, and predisposing/ precipitating/perpetuating factors. Then follows a mental state examination, risk assessment, physical examination, and appropriate physical and social investigations. Collateral information is gathered from relatives and friends. Mental state examination is essentially the same as that for younger adults, with particular attention to the mood, presence of suicidal ideas and cognitive assessment. Standardized assessment scales, including the Mini-Mental State Examination (MMSE), Abbreviated Mental Test (AMT) and the short form of the Geriatric Depression Scale (GDS) are commonly used. The Hamilton Depression Rating Scale is also used occasionally. Chinese versions of the above scales are available and are locally validated. A risk assessment includes self-harm and depression-related self-neglect. The former is particularly relevant given the very high rate of suicide in the elderly in Hong Kong.

Management

Miss LC would be managed in either an inpatient or outpatient setting depending on factors such as the severity of depression, suicidal risk and adequacy of social support.

Her coexisting physical health problems, disabilities and pain associated with COPD and osteoarthritis will be alleviated as far as possible. Social care needs will be addressed, and support from relatives and community resources mobilized. Non-pharmacological treatment such as psycho-education and supportive counselling are commonly administered by the doctor or other professionals such as mental health nurses. Cognitive behaviour therapy (CBT) or psychological interventions will be considered where appropriate.

Antidepressant drug treatment is usually prescribed for patients with moderate to severe depression. Hong Kong has a brief guideline on the management of depression for psychiatrists. First-line antidepressants include a tricyclic, a tetracyclic or a selective serotonin reuptake inhibitor (SSRI). In the older persons like Miss LC an SSRI is usually the preferred option. Other newer antidepressants like serotonin norepinephrine reuptake inhibitors (SNRI) and noradrenergic and specific serotonergic antidepressants (NaSSA) are also used in older adults. Electroconvulsive therapy (ECT) is reserved for depressed elderly who are actively suicidal, or require a rapid response because of risks to health.

Barriers to effective treatment

In Hong Kong, depression is still an under-recognized and under-treated disorder. The main barriers to effective treatment include the following: stigma associated with mental health problems; lack of public awareness; ageism; misconceptions about depression and its treatment; and the long waiting time (up to six months) in psychiatric clinics within the public sector. In addition, the recent outbreaks of infectious diseases like severe acute respiratory syndrome (SARS) and avian flu have led to a shift of priorities by government and the public, with resources now targeted less on mental health and towards infectious disease control. Hence, detection and treatment of depression and suicide prevention in the older persons would remain a major challenge in Hong Kong.

REFERENCES

Chiu H. F. K., Pang A. H. T., Lam L. C. W. (1996) Letter from Hong Kong. *Int. J. Geriatr. Psychiatry* **11**, 711–13.

Chiu H. F. K., Takahashi Y, Suh G. H. (2003) Elderly suicide prevention in East Asia. *Int. J. Geriatr. Psychiatry* **18**, 973–6.

Japan

Dr Syuichi Awata, Psychiatrist and Director, Division of Neuropsychiatry and Center for Dementia, Sendai City Hospital, and Dr Akira Honma, Psychiatrist, Tokyo Metropolitan Institute of Gerontology

Presentation

Patients like Miss LC are frequent in practice in Japan but unlike this patient, most older people live in their own homes rather than in an assisted-living facility. Even so, many elderly women experience loneliness after losing their husbands or because of a lack of communication with a living spouse and/or other family members. The presence of physical illness and/or disability is very likely to contribute feelings of helplessness, hopelessness, and worthlessness. Poor physical health and social isolation are risk factors for depression in the elderly and together with depression are independently associated with self-harm and suicide in older adults in Japan and other cultures (Conwell *et al.* 2002, O'Connell *et al.* 2005).

Miss LC presents with symptoms typical of depressive disorder including fatigue, low energy, sleep disturbance, irritability, feeling miserable and thoughts of death. Chronic pain and shortness of breath will exacerbate depression in this case and depression itself may increase the intensity of both symptoms via a vicious cycle between physical and psychological symptoms. Depression is often unrecognized in community and primary care settings. This is because older depressed people often stay indoors because they are depressed, reducing the likelihood of consulting and because primary care physicians and those close to the patient are often not familiar with the symptoms of depression. Because depression is linked to poorer health outcomes and suicide, much more work is needed in Japan to educate the community and primary care physicians about diagnosis and treatment of late-life depression.

Assessment

I strongly recommend that community mental health professionals and primary care physicians use a brief scale in order to more easily detect depressive disorders and assess symptom severity, risk of suicide, and health-related quality of life of elderly depressed patients. One option is the WHO-Five Well-Being Index (WHO-5) (World Health Organization 2005). Since each item concerns positive well-being, health-care professionals are willing to use it and elderly community residents are likely to accept it. The scale has been translated into various languages and validated in the context of various health states, including depressive disorders (Bonsignore *et al.* 2001, Henkel *et al.* 2003, 2004), anxiety disorders (Bonsignore *et al.* 2001), psychiatric disorders (Heun *et al.* 1999), and health-related quality of life (Bech *et al.* 2003). It has good psychometric properties in older depressed patients (Heun *et al.* 1999). Bonsignore *et al.* (2001) reported that the second version of the WHO-5 performs well in detecting depressive disorders in elderly primary care patients. It has been also suggested that the WHO-5 might be helpful for preventing suicide through improved patient management of depression (Hegerl and Althaus 2003). The Japanese version of the WHO-5 has also been validated in the context of detecting depressive disorders in diabetic patients (Awata *et al.* 2007a) and suicidal ideation in the general elderly population (Awata *et al.* 2007b).

A geriatric psychiatrist would diagnose her symptoms as a major or minor depressive disorder according to DSM-IV or ICD-10. Symptom severity is usually assessed using the Hamilton Rating Scale for Depression or the Montgomery Äsberg Depression Rating Scale. The risk for suicide is also assessed on the basis of the knowledge obtained from the studies on risk factors for suicide in elderly people. In this case, chronic obstructive pulmonary disease (COPD), chronic pain (Quan *et al.* 2002) and lack of social support (Awata *et al.* 2005a) would be regarded as increasing this risk and would be taken into account in Miss LC's management.

An important nationwide social system to detect elderly depressed people in Japan is the community welfare volunteer, 'Minsei-iin', comprising individuals appointed in each community by the Minister of Health and Welfare for three-year terms. Their aim is to understand community needs and liaise with welfare offices and other community resources. Community welfare volunteers can be the first to identify distressed older people in which case they trigger a visit by a community nurse to evaluate depression and suicide risk.

Management

After such an assessment, psychosocial treatment would be initiated and that would be the case with Miss LC. An outreach programme that includes depression case management might be one way that support is provided. Under this programme, community nurses are educated to provide problem-solving therapy to elderly depressed people in the community. A community nurse regularly visits the client's home, for example two-weekly. The approach is to use attentive and empathic listening skills in order form a therapeutic alliance sufficient to clarify concerns and focus on which problems to address. Support is provided by psychiatrists and the community mental health team. If necessary the latter may also plan and implement specialist care in collaboration with primary care. This approach has been shown to improve well-being and reduce suicidal ideation in elderly depressed people living in an urban residential district (Awata *et al.* 2005b).

Selective serotonin reuptake inhibitors (SSRIs) such as paroxetine, fluvoxamine and sertraline are recommended first-line drug treatments. Selective serotonin and noradrenaline reuptake inhibitors (SNRIs), for example milnacipram, and other antidepressants (trazodone, mianserine, nortriptyline, maprotyline and amoxapine) are also used in patients for whom SSRIs are unsuitable or poorly tolerated. Electroconvulsive therapy (ECT) might also be considered for patients who have medication resistance or intolerance and/ or for those who need rapid improvement due to severe mental and/or physical health conditions.

The Japan Medical Association published *The Manual for Suicide Prevention* in 2004, which provides a guideline for primary care physicians in the diagnosis and treatment of depression. As a geriatric psychiatrist I can offer support to primary care physicians in the diagnosis, treatment and management of geriatric psychiatric patients. The biggest barrier to effective treatment of elderly depressed patients in our health-care system is the extreme shortage of geriatric psychiatrists and mental health professionals, despite the fact that Japan is now facing an unprecedented rapid growth of an ageing population.

REFERENCES

Awata S., Seki T., Koizumi Y., *et al.* (2005a) Factors associated with suicidal ideation in an elderly urban Japanese population: a community-based cross-sectional study. *Psychiatr. Clin. Neurosci.* **59**, 327–36.

Awata S., Seki T., Koizumi Y., *et al.* (2005b) Effects of a comprehensive community intervention model to reduce late-life depression and suicidal ideation in an urban residential district. *Int. Psychogeriatrics* **17** (Suppl. 2), 381–2.

Awata S., Bech P., Yoshida S., *et al.* (2007a). Reliability and validity of the Japanese version of the WHO-Five Well-Being Index in the context of detecting depression in diabetic patients. *Psychiatr. Clin. Neurosci.* **61**, 112–19.

Awata S., Bech P., Koizumi Y., *et al.* (2007b). Validity and utility of the Japanese version of the WHO-Five Well-Being Index in the context of detecting suicidal ideation in elderly community residents. *Int. Psychogeriatrics* **19**, 77–88.

Bech P., Olsen L. R., Kjoller M., Rasmussen, N. K. (2003) Measuring well-being rather than the absence of distress symptoms: a comparison of the SF-36 Mental Health subscale and the WHO-Five Well-Being Scale. *Int. J. Methods Psychiatr. Res.* **12**, 85–91.

Bonsignore M., Barkow K., Jessen F., Heun R. (2001) Validity of the five-item WHO Well-Being Index (WHO-5) in an elderly population. *Eur. Arch. Psychiatry Clin. Neurosci.* **251** (Suppl. 2), II/27–II/31.

Conwell Y., Duberstein P. R., Caine E. (2002) Risk factors for suicide in later life. *Biol. Psychiatry* **52**, 193–204.

Hegerl U., Althaus D. (2003) From patient screening to management list in suicide risk: practical guidelines for dealing with depression. *MMW Fortshritte der Medizin*, **145**: 24–27.

Henkel V., Mergl R., Kohnen R., *et al.* (2003) Identifying depression in primary care: a comparison of different methods in a prospective cohort study. *Br. Med. J.* **326**, 200–1.

Henkel V., Mergl R., Coynbe J. C., *et al.* (2004) Screening for depression in primary care: will one or two items suffice? *Eur. Arch. Psychiatry Clin. Neurosci.* **254**, 215–23.

Heun R., Burkart M., Maier M., Bech P. (1999) Internal and external validity of the WHO Well-Being Scale in the elderly general population. *Acta Psychiatr. Scand.* **99**, 171–8.

Japan Medical Association (2004) *The Manual for Suicide Prevention.* Tokyo: Japan Medical Association.

O'Connell H., Chin A. V., Cunningham C., Lawlor B. (2005). Recent developments: suicide in older people. *Br. Med. J.* **329**, 895–9.

Quan H., Arboleda-Florez J., Fick G. H., *et al.* (2002) Association between physical illness and suicide among the elderly. *Soc. Psychiatry Psychiatr. Epidemiol.* **37**, 190–7.

World Health Organization (2005) *WHO-Five Well-Being Index.* Geneva: WHO. Available online at www.who-5.org/

The Netherlands

Dr Els Licht-Strunk, General Practitioner, VU University Medical Centre, Amsterdam, and Dr Marijke Bremmer, Consultant Psychiatrist, VU University Medical Centre, Amsterdam

The Dutch health-care system

In the Netherlands, all patients are registered with a general practitioner (GP) who acts as a gate-keeper, which means that patients need a referral for specialized mental health care. In our health-care system, older people can get help from home nurses for assistance in household and activities of daily living (ADL). Institutionalized care for older people is organized in residential homes and nursing homes. Although both resident groups need help in daily life because of physical or cognitive impairments, residents in nursing homes are more in need of help with ADL activities than those in residential homes. Medical care for people living in residential homes is delivered by GPs, whereas in nursing homes medical care is provided by especially trained nursing home physicians who have completed a two-year postgraduate academic education.

Medical problems of patients living in residential homes are discussed with the GP. Older patients can contact the GP by themselves and ask for a home visit, for they are often not able to visit the practice. It is also possible that one of the nurses or relatives contact the GP for a medical question. Furthermore, some GPs arrange visits to the residents on a regular basis, for example every two or three months, either carried out by themselves or by their practice nurses. This helps being proactive in patients with multi-morbidity and solving problems in an early stage.

Guidelines

Our Dutch Society of General Practice has published about 90 guidelines on conditions frequently seen in general practice. These guidelines are widely accepted and used by most of the GPs. One of them is on depression (Van Marwijk *et al.* 2003). About 90% of all depressed patients are treated in primary care. The depression guideline presents a list with the nine symptoms of depressive disorder according to the DSM-IV. GPs are recommended to use these when they suspect a case of depression, but they are not encouraged to screen for depression in high-risk groups. The guideline also gives advice on treatment, but does not have a specific section aimed at the geriatric population.

Access to specialist psychiatric care is always through the GP. This system requires good collaboration between the two parties with respect to the individual patient but also with respect to organizing adequate psychiatric care at a regional level. For instance, psychiatric nurses working in ambulatory care settings are being posted as consultants at the practice of a GP one day a week. This is being done to support the GP in recognizing and treating 'minor' psychiatric illnesses such as non-suicidal depression, anxiety disorders and somatization. This system is also believed to lower the threshold for referral to psychiatric care, when needed. For older patients, adequate collaboration between the two parties is even more important. Often, GPs are quite well informed about the family situation. Especially in geriatric psychiatry, physical diseases, emotional problems and the patient's social situation are inseparable domains and in each case interventions need to be geared to one another.

Assessment by the GP

Miss LC lives in a residential home and I am her GP. She has a complex medical history with her multi-morbidity of osteoarthritis and chronic obstructive pulmonary disease (COPD) and is probably taking several drugs. As she is feeling tired and miserable, often not bothering to answer the telephone, I don't expect her to come to me with a clear request for help. Probably one of the nurses or relatives calls me to ask me to come by, because they are worried about this lady. I have known Miss LC for a couple of years now and I have seen her deteriorate. Both conditions are progressive and her disability is getting worse. It is very reasonable that this makes her feel sad. I will make an appointment to visit her.

When I see Miss LC she looks depressed and sad. When I ask her how she feels, she starts complaining about her pains in the knees and back and the shortness of breath. She is frustrated that she stopped smoking ages ago, and still this emphysema is getting worse. She is increasingly dependent on the nurses. Sometimes the pain and breathlessness are so bad that she can't get out of bed to go to the toilet at night. Recently she wet herself, because the nurse she called for came in too late. 'Life is of no use for me like this, doctor,' she says, and starts crying.

I will ask what Miss LC thinks I can do for her. During our conversation I would try to find out whether she is having a depressive disorder and especially whether she has suicidal ideations or plans. Before considering treatment for depression, I would first pay more attention to her somatic problems. What medication is she taking? Can her symptoms have got worse due to side effects or polypharmacy? How is her COPD being treated? What painkillers is she taking? Can these treatments be optimized? Is the breathlessness really due to the respiratory problem, or has she for example developed a heart failure? After all, heart failure is often not recognized in patients with COPD and its symptoms can increase when using non-steroidal anti-inflammatory drugs (NSAIDs), which she is probably taking for her osteoarthritis. I would do a physical examination and I would like to do some blood tests on her, especially to rule out anaemia and hypothyroidism.

I would talk with Miss LC about what she wants. Are there any activities she enjoyed and has stopped doing? If so, I would try with her to identify barriers which have made her stop doing them. For example, is she not going to the weekly lunch at the church because she doesn't want to, or because she doesn't know how to get there? Assuming that the suicide risk is low, I would end my visit here. I will arrange the blood tests by asking a laboratory assistant to visit her. And I will ask Miss LC to think about activities that she might want to start doing (again) which can help her feel better.

The next week, I will visit Miss LC again. The blood results have not shown an explanation for her mood problems or breathlessness. She has not come up with a list of activities she wants to do. I would ask Miss LC whether she agrees that I invite a psychiatrist or psychiatric nurse to come and visit her. Because of the multi-morbidity, disability and problem with interactions due to her polypharmacy I would like to get advice from a specialist from the department of geriatric psychiatry.

If Miss LC had been suicidal at my first visit, I would have made a referral to the psychiatrist that same day.

The role of the psychiatrist

Miss LC may have been referred to me by the psychiatric nurse, being consultant of the residential home, or by the GP.

Some very important aspects of her history have been given, but there is not yet any clue as to why we think she became clinically depressed (anhedonia, sleep problems with early awakening, tiredness, irritability and worthlessness) at this moment. This is important because it may help us find an adequate treatment. More history needs to be taken. How does she recognize her situation? Why does she think life is not worth living? Does she think that her pain and breathlessness are causing her feelings? How about her social life: how does she relate to the staff and to the other residents? Could she be mourning over the loss of a friend or a family member? Also, has she been depressed earlier in her life? If so, what has helped her before? And what did not do so?

Probably her GP knows her well and consultation about her psychiatric history and her current somatic condition is important.

Therapeutic options

In the Netherlands, guidelines for the treatment of depression include both biological therapies and talking therapies (Netherlands Institute of Mental Health and Addiction 2005). By law, mental health care is accessible and free for all residents. However there is some restriction to talking therapies with a limit of 25 sessions for Axis I disorders and 50 sessions for Axis II disorders. Although there are no financial barriers for anyone, depressive disorders, especially in the elderly, are under-treated and probably under-recognized. Epidemiological data show that only 20% of the elderly fulfilling criteria for major depression are treated with antidepressants, while 40% receive benzodiazepines. Between 10% and 25% were receiving formal mental health care (Beekman *et al.* 1997).

In the case of Miss LC, there are some clues that supportive therapy or cognitive therapy may be helpful. Especially inter-personal psychotherapy (IPT) may be helpful if we think that her depression arose within a context of inter-personal loss, such as a dispute with a friend of family member, a role transition (moving from independent housing to residential care), grief or inter-personal deficits (such as social impoverishment). IPT has proven to be practical and effective in geriatric depression (van Schaik *et al.* 2006). Since this is a manual-based psychotherapy, it can be given both by psychotherapists and by trained nurses.

If we think that her depressive behaviour has impaired her ability to relate to the staff, some guidance to them, and instructions towards the patient, may clear the air. Probably this patient will need some encouragement from the staff to prevent her from isolating herself. This should be done in a non-judgemental manner, with respect for her autonomy and with mutual consent.

Next to talking therapies, pharmacotherapy is an important component of depression treatment in the elderly, even with co-morbid conditions. In severe or even psychotic depressive disorders, antidepressants are the first therapeutic option. In general, doctors are reluctant to prescribe antidepressants to the elderly and if they do, often the dosage is too low. With this patient, the antidepressant of first choice would be the one that has been proven to be safe and effective for her previously. Otherwise the Dutch guidelines (Netherlands Institute of Mental Health and Addiction 2006) recommend starting with a selective serotonin reuptake inhibitor (SSRI) with minimal pharmacological interactions. If Miss LC appears to be very seriously depressed and suicidal or psychotic, it is advisable to start with tricyclic antidepressants immediately, sometimes even with electroconvulsive therapy (ECT).

There is also an important safety aspect to her depression. The prevalence of suicide increases with age, especially after 50, although more in men than in women. We will need to evaluate her suicidality. Does she consider suicide as an option? Does she have a plan on how to end her life? Does she have access to lethal substances? Besides depression, important risk factors for suicide are previous attempts, agitation, impulsivity, psychosis and substance abuse. I will evaluate this aspect of her depression with her, and if necessary take precautions. Temporary admission to a psychiatric ward is always an option when the risk of suicide cannot be managed outside.

So, different ways to manage her depression are at hand. Evidence favours a combined treatment of any form of psychotherapy and pharmacotherapy. According to Dutch law, Miss LC will have to be informed about the diagnosis, her treatment options and possible harmful effects, and she will have to consent to the treatment protocol. When the active depression has been treated and if Miss LC's future needs are for maintenance pharmacotherapy solely, then referring her back to the GP is a reasonable option.

REFERENCES

Beekman A. T. F., Deeg D., Braam A. W., Smit J. H., van Tilburg W. (1997) Consequences of major and minor depression in later life: a study of disability, well-being and service utilization. *Psychol. Med.* **27**, 1397–409.

Netherlands Institute of Mental Health and Addiction (2006) *Multidisciplinaire Richtlijn Depressie* [Multidisciplinary Guidelines for the Treatment of Depression]:, *Addendum for Late-Life Depression.* Utrecht: Trimbos Institut.

Van Marwijk H., Grundmeijer H., Bijl D., *et al.* (2003) *NHG-Standaard Depressieve Stoornis (Depressie)*, Eerste herziening. [Dutch College of General Practitioners Guideline Depression, first revision] *Huisarts Wet.* **46**, 614–33.

van Schaik D. J. F., van Marwijk H., Ader H., *et al.* (2006) Interpersonal psychotherapy for elderly patients in primary care. *Am. J. Geriatr. Psychiatry* **14**, 777–86.

Norway

Professor Knut Engedal, Professor of Old-Age Psychiatry, Ullevaal University Hospital, Oslo, and Professor Harald Sanaker, Specialist in Family Medicine, Kongsvegen Legesenter, Brummunddal

Norwegian health-care system

Until recently, the public health-care system has been the only professional health service in Norway. The private market for health service is now growing, but most health service is still provided by public funding. Norway has a three-tier system for the provision of public health and social care based on the Municipal Health Care Act, the Social Care Act, the Hospital Act and the National Insurance Act. Local authorities are responsible for the patient list system, whereas the state is responsible for the specialist health-care service, including the hospitals. Every general practitioner (GP) is responsible for a defined segment of the population in a patient list system. GPs act as gate-keepers of the health-care system.

Assessment

In the Norwegian system Miss LC would therefore see her GP first. It is likely that the GP would initiate management and treatment of both her somatic disorders and her depression. The GP would use a holistic approach when assessing Miss LC's health status. Before starting treatment for depression the GP would assess Miss LC's symptoms due to chronic obstructive pulmonary disease (COPD) and pain due to osteoarthritis and aim to optimally manage these problems. Thereafter, the GP needs to assess Miss LC's symptoms of depression by a detailed history exploring depressive symptoms. Some GPs will use questions taken from a standardized instrument like Montgomery Åsberg Rating Scale (MADRAS) or the Geriatric Depression Scale (GDS) and some would even use the instrument in its entirety. The MADRAS is most likely to be use in Miss LC's case partly because it is very popular and partly because GPs are paid extra (as part of their contract) for using it.

Management

If the GP thinks that Miss LC has a depressive disorder (and the score is above 15 and below 36 on MADRAS) antidepressant treatment should be discussed with the patient and initiated. If the score is above 35 or if Miss LC expresses suicidal thoughts she should be referred to specialist health-care immediately. If the patient is severely depressed and has delusions, electroconvulsive therapy (ECT) will for some patients be the first-line treatment at specialist care level. For others, treatment with antidepressants should first be offered.

First-line treatment is usually a selective serotonin reuptake inhibitor (SSRI) or perhaps mianserin in view of Miss LC's sleep difficulties. Although non-selective monamine reuptake inhibitors such as amitryptyline will have some effect on her pain, they would not normally be first-line because of Miss LC's age and because of anticholinergic effects (often reducing compliance) and risk of drug interaction and toxicity. The GP will also encourage Miss LC to visit the communal room in her sheltered accommodation and to rejoin the lunch group at her church. Behavioural activation can be a useful strategy that the GP can utilize. In addition he or she will offer to see Miss LC regularly, perhaps on a weekly basis at the start of treatment and every second week later on. The purpose of these consultations will be to titrate the drug treatment, to support Miss LC and to encourage her to resume activities that she has previously found enjoyable.

If the depression does not improve within two months the GP would usually consider trying another drug, either a different SSRI, mianserin (if not pre-scribed initially), mirtazapine–venlafaxine (dual acting), or reboxetine (nor-adrenaline specific). If this is not successful the GP will ask for advice from a specialist in psychiatry (via the telephone) or refer Miss LC to an outpatient clinic either in adult psychiatry or in old-age psychiatry. Access to the latter in major cities is good. The local district nurse will be asked to bring in services that could address Miss LC's loneliness, or refer her to a day centre for old people affiliated to a local nursing home. Day centres can provide up to three meals a day, social and occupational activities, and transport to the centre and return to the patient's home. Local authorities cover most of the costs so Miss LC would pay little. Whether someone like Miss LC with protracted symptoms of depression will be referred to a day centre will depend on local resources. In all Norwegian municipalities psychiatric nurses can provide services to psychi-atric patients but in some areas it is limited and younger patients and patients with chronic psychiatric disorders are often prioritized. The specialist psychia-trist in some cases offers psychotherapy, or works together with a psychologist who can offer time-limited psychotherapy, although this is not available in all areas.

Admission

If depression still persists, Miss LC will be admitted to inpatient treatment in a department of old-age psychiatry which are available in parts of the country. Here treatment will combine various elements such as drugs, ECT, social activities and support, with encouragement of involvement by family members. After discharge, some elderly patients will be followed up by the outpatient clinic either in adult psychiatry or old-age psychiatry, but all will need to be followed up by their GP. The treatment will be continued for at least six months after recovery in patients with a first episode of depression, and for longer in patients with recurrent depression. The GP plays an important role in encouraging the patient to continue to take their medication as well as identifying relapse after the medication has been stopped.

Romania

Dr Nicoleta Tătaru, Senior Consultant Psychiatrist, Forensic Hospital Ştei, Bihor, Dr Monica Bălan, Primary Care Physician, Oradea, and Dr Alexandru Dicker, Senior Consultant in Internal Medicine, Psychiatric Hospital Nucet, Bihor

Mental health-care system in Romania

Romania is a developing former Communist country in Eastern Europe with a population of 21 794 793 (2002) covering 237 500 km^2. Fourteen per cent of the general population are over the age of 65.

Most psychiatric services are provided by hospitals and outpatient services of the Ministry of Health. As is historically true of other countries, the special needs of mentally ill people were not always recognized and respected by the generic services. Stigma remains an obstacle in ensuring access to good care for mentally ill patients. In relation to patients' needs and quality of life, standards need to be raised in basic mental health care.

Only recently has Romania developed community mental health-care services, alongside the traditional system of psychiatric hospital care. Mental health legislation only appeared in Romania in August 2002 (Government of Romania 2002). This was the first step towards reform of the mental health services and care system of mentally ill patients.

A national mental health programme has developed in recent years for the treatment of schizophrenia and depression, to provide free medication for the patients when diagnosed and for inpatients in forensic psychiatric units. The national programme for care of the elderly is still only a project in that currently it is lacking financial support.

In 2003 a programme for residential care and after-care of patients started, including for older patients with mental disorders and dementia (Health Department 2003). There is some financial support from the Labour Department and Social Protection too as a compensation for families or care-givers of the chronically ill with a handicap (including those with dementia), who are treated at their home. To involve general practitioners (GPs) and community nurses in the care of the elderly we have initiated an educational programme.

Caring for the mentally ill elderly requires an understanding of biological changes in late life and how late-life mental disorders specifically present. It also requires skills to recognize medical co-morbidity in older depressed people and an understanding of the high prevalence of depression and the cognitive and non-cognitive symptoms of dementia. As in other parts of the world, we believe that old-age mental illnesses are under-recognized and under-treated. Unfortunately, we do not have either a clear picture of all services for elderly care.

Presentation

In Romania, Miss LC would present to the GP. He or she will treat the patient and after one to three weeks the GP may send her to the ambulatory internal medicine specialist. This practitioner may recommend admission to a general hospital for relief of somatic symptoms.

However, in Romania, such patients often end up in psychiatric services because their multiple complaints are taken by the physicians to represent psychiatric symptoms.

Only a proportion of patients like Miss LC with physical co-morbidity are recognized by GPs as depressed. Only around 30% of depressed patients are diagnosed by GPs and referred to the psychiatrists. Depression is common alongside other psychiatric disorders (anxiety, personality disorders, dementia, drugs, polypharmacology and alcoholism), as well as with physical disorders like those of Miss LC. Chronic physical illnesses increase dependence on others, cause chronic pain and discomfort and reduce mobility. In our country depressed patients can suffer with one of several types: major depression with early onset and late onset, with or without psychotic symptoms, depression with or without cognitive impairment (pseudo-dementia), chronic dysthymia, neurotic depression, organic depression, vascular depression. We have to be particularly watchful for patients who come to us with depression as the first symptom of dementia.

Epidemiological studies in this field are lacking in Romania. We encourage practitioners to be aware that minor depression with physical co-morbidity is common and significant and not a trivial problem.

It is important to have a high index of suspicion of depression, particularly in people with poor health who have low mood, impaired cognition, low motivation, loneliness and present pain.

To assess older depressed patients we use the 4-item Geriatric Depression Scale (GDS) in primary care and the 15- and 30-item GDS and Hamilton Rating Scale of Depression in psychiatric wards.

The principal risk factors for depression in Romania are as elsewhere: reduced social networks, loneliness, bereavement, poverty, physical ill health, poor self-esteem, lack of capacity for intimacy and genetic factors. All have to be evaluated with all elderly patients. To assess the most important risk, suicide, the practitioners undertake a complete clinical, psychiatric and psychological examination and will usually admit the patient to a closed ward with early treatment with antidepressants, sedation, anxiolytics, electroconvulsive therapy (ECT) and psychotherapy.

Management

Thus, the first steps in the management of this patient will be: the treatment of chronic obstructive pulmonary disease with anticholinergic bronchodilatators, beta-2 long-term agonist, antibiotics, long-term oxygen therapy, pain management with analgesics, kinetotherapy and psychotherapy.

Depression in an older patient with co-morbidity such as Miss LC will be treated with a newer antidepressant such as a selective serotonin reuptake inhibitor (SSRI), a serotonin norepinephrine reuptake inhibitor (SNRI) (dual-uptake drugs) or noradrenaline reuptake inhibitor (NaRI). These newer drugs are effective, safe and we find can improve also poor cognitive functioning linked to depression. We recommend treatment for at least 12 months for major depression.

In Romania we do not have any depression protocols or guidelines as yet. Pharmacotherapy is not the only treatment modality in late-life depression in Romania. Psychotherapy is also available to some patients. Nowadays, in Romania GPs increasingly also use complementary medicine.

In addition to the traditional system of acute hospital care, community care allows a variety of treatment options to be provided in the person's own home, including day care centres or other care-provider services. By these means we aim to improve quality of life in frailer old depressed patients. Psychiatrists collaborate with GPs, internal medicine specialists and psychotherapists, social workers and other care-provider services and are usually responsible for the initial treatment plan for depression, using the combined treatment (medication and psychotherapy).

The most important barriers to effective treatment of depressed patients in our health-care system are the under-recognition of mental disorders and the stigma and discrimination in treating them. Stigma and discrimination are thus special problems in late-life mental health problems, including depression. Recognition of depression by GPs is another problem and depends on their awareness of how the ageing process affects the presentation of depressive disorder and whether they give equal weight to physical and mental health. GPs remain the gatekeepers. Multiple losses in old age, social isolation and loneliness are among the most frequent latent causes of hospitalization and of placement in nursing homes.

In conclusion, as elsewhere older depressed patients present with co-morbidity, either physical, cognitive or both, and would benefit from complex rehabilitation programmes with more substantial social and financial support from the government and local authorities and with input from users and care-givers. Community care centres require further development as an alternative to hospitalization. The place of non-pharmacological treatments has not been adequately investigated but they are part of the 'complete management pack-age' in late-life mental disorders. Finally, there is need to focus on improving the quality of life of frail and mentally ill elderly living in nursing and residential settings.

REFERENCES

Government of Romania (2002) Mental Health Law. *Monitorul oficial al Romaniei* **XIV**(589), August 2002.

Health Department (2003) Standards for residence care. *Monitorul oficial al Romaniei*, **XV**(255), April 2003.

Spain

Professor Raimundo Mateos, Professor of Psychiatry, University of Santiago de Compostela, and Dr Jose Antonio Ferreiro Guri, Specialist in Family and Community Medicine, University of Santiago de Compostela

Spanish health-care system

In Spain, the National Health System covers virtually the whole of the pop-ulation. Every citizen is assigned a general practitioner (GP), and Miss LC would initially be seen by a GP at the local health centre or, if relevant, a doctor contracted to the sheltered accommodation where she lives.

Presentation of depression

In Spain, publications and forums on primary health care point to a wide-spread under-diagnosis of depressive disorder (Perez-Franco and Turabian-Fernandez 2006). Lack of time and the tendency of older depressed patients in particular to somatize may initially make diagnosis difficult for the GP. Patients attending primary health care verbalize emotional disorders less frequently than consultations specifically for mental health problems. Nevertheless, whether by intuition or a few well-directed questions, as soon as a background of emotional distress is revealed, GPs can make time to re-interview the patient in better circumstances (the so-called 'organized' or 'arranged' surgery at specific times). Miss LC's case is a good example of the need for additional surgery time (Cerecedo-Pérez and Ruiz-Gómes 2005). The first priority of the GP is likely to be to deal with the biological causes of physical complaints, checking the progress of the physical illness in the face of apparent worsening of functional impairment and its emotional repercussions, or new symptoms that suggest an additional health problem. This would call for an adequate history supplemented where possible by objective instruments such as analogue scales of pain, stage of dyspnoea, etc., in order to monitor the physical symptoms. Physical examination, including a neurological examination, would follow. Investigations such as an erythrocyte sedimentation rate (ESR), haemoglobin, biochemical profile including tests of renal and hepatic function, thyroid hormones and vitamin B_{12} would be ordered to rule physical diseases that might not have been detected (for example, thyroid dysfunction, heart failure, malignancy). Other tests, depending on the presentation, may include an electrocardiogram (ECG), radiology (in this case of the chest) and spirometry (Von Korff et al. 2002).

Miss LC's case reveals a number of risk factors for depression: female gender, older age, loss of family links and loss of physical functions. In turn these may interact with stressful life events which may further affect her mood. Even so, when and how was the current situation triggered? How long has she lived in the supervised accommodation? How does she experience life in the supervised accommodation? Have conflicts arisen? Does she have friends? Have there been any family bereavements recently? Has she had a previous history of depression? Markers of 'frailty' (to be understood here as a risk of progressive functional deterioration, dependency and death), a risk factor for depression, should be identified: recent admissions to hospital, polypharmacy, visual and/ or hearing complaints, recent falls, low body mass index, cognitive impairment, incontinence and so forth (Peveler et al. 2002). Miss LC has a number of symptoms which add up to a depressive disorder: emotional symptoms (apathy, feeling miserable); cognitive symptoms (pessimism, feelings of guilt, self-reproach, hopelessness); behavioural (decreased interest in habitual activities, isolation) and somatic preoccupations (myalgia, breathing difficulties, changes in sleeping pattern).

Assessment

Interest in the diagnosis and treatment of depression in primary care has increased enormously over the last decade. In Spain, the reasons have more to do with information and training efforts by the pharmaceutical industry than to any formal co-ordination between specialized mental health networks and primary care. Seminars on and clinical trials of new antidepressants in primary care have helped GPs become familiar with screening tools and clinical scales of depression, as well as with diagnostic criteria from ICD-10 and DSM-IV (Mateos et al. 2001). The use of the Geriatric Depression Scale (GDS) seems to be preferred for elderly people (Fernandez-San Martin *et al.* 2002); however, it is debatable as to how routinely these are used in busy practice. Nor does the use of a screening tool obviate the need for a detailed case history. In Miss LC's case an assessment of the risk of suicide should be added.

Management

Having ruled out other possible 'organic' disorders by history, examination and complementary tests, the next step is management. One of the causes of 'failure' of antidepressants is that the patient does not take the medication properly. Therefore the doctor–patient relation becomes particularly important. This includes aspects of empathy, exploration of beliefs, fears and resistances, a shared choice of a therapeutic option, easily understandable information on what will happen, and side effects. The choice of antidepressant is determined by what best suits the patient, in other words it is tailored to her situation although realistically it must be one the GP is familiar with using. Initially because of its tolerance, safety profile and long experience in use, we would probably opt for a selective serotonin reuptake inhibitor (SSRI), and given that Miss LC shows apathy, the choice of fluoxetine could be indicated for its disinhibitory effect. Because of her age, the initial dosage will be half that recommended for younger adults. It may take up to six weeks for full therapeutic effect, during which time the dose may be increased. Her sleeping problems should be addressed by a sleep hygiene approach, with timetables prescribing moderate physical activity, bedtime and awakening time, not napping and avoiding hypnotic drugs.

Given the multifactorial nature of depression (emotional, cognitive and behavioural) not all may respond to pharmacotherapy. Apart from the support provided by the medical practice by encouraging understanding what depression is, building self-confidence and helping put things in perspective, in primary care brief psychotherapy is often recommended, which can maximize therapeutic benefit in the very short time usually available (Tizón 1996).

A team approach

If Miss LC presented to our locality, she would have the benefit of a team which is located in an urban health centre where specialists in Family and Community Medicine work within a multidisciplinary team of nurses and a social worker. Also, the centre has had the support of the only unit for psychogeriatrics in Galicia for more than a decade, with a monthly visit by a psychogeriatrician. This means that it is easier for us than other areas of Spain to comply with the maxims we have outlined above and that there is a clear need for initiatives nationally to improve multidisciplinary practice and the relations between these two levels of health care (Tizón 1996).

Barriers to treatment

Probably one of the greatest obstacles primary care teams must surmount is lack of awareness about depressive disorder. Natural motivation and a personal effort by primary care doctors to squeeze in some time to devote to a whole range of diagnostic challenges, including emotional disorders, are determiners. Pressures on primary health care, the varying levels of motivation of GPs, their natural aptitude or otherwise to address emotional problems in a complex case, congestion in the mental health units which make even more urgent referrals difficult, the high prevalence of these diseases and the ensuing demand for follow-up visits all act as barriers. With 40–50 patients to see and five minutes for each, there is a temptation to skip an open question which may reveal depression or simply to keep silent. A lack of training in and availability of structured psychotherapeutic alternatives poses a serious problem (Tellez-Lapeira *et al.* 2005). A suitable structured brief psychotherapy service in primary care would require at least 20 minutes per session per week for around three months per patient. This might though be more productive than a series of five minute appointments which achieve little.

Even with the best clinical guidelines or protocols, the management of emotional problems which coexist with physical disorders poses the physician a much greater challenge than when presented in isolation. In these cases, the art of healing must always take priority over the science. Expertly put: 'Yet a humane and balanced approach to care frequently leads to an appreciable improvement in the well-being of the older adult suffering a chronic, even fatal illness' (Blazer 1998).

REFERENCES

Blazer D. (1998) Emotional problems associated with physical illness. In *Emotional Problems in Later Life: Intervention Strategies for Professional Caregivers*, 2nd edn. New York: Springer, pp. 181–99.

Cerecedo-Pérez M.J., Ruiz-Gómes M. (2005) Abordaje de los problemas de salud mental: 'Doctora estoy deprimida.' – Abordaje de las alteraciones del estado de ánimo por el médico de familia [The management of mental health problems: 'Doctor I am depressed.' – The management of mood disorders by the family doctor]. *Formación Acreditada On-Line: El Médico Interactivo*. Available online at www.elmedicointeractivo.com/formacion_acre2005/temas/tema5-6/abordaje.htm.

Fernandez-San Martin M.I., Andrade C., Molina J., *et al.* (2002) Validation of the Spanish version of the Geriatric Depression Scale (GDS) in primary care. *Int. J. Geriatr. Psychiatry* **17**, 279–87.

Mateos R., Gómez-Campos R. (2001) Diagnóstico y tratamiento de la ansiedad en el anciano, Serie Grandes Síndromes Geriatricos. *Protocolos de la Sociedad Española de Geriatría y Gerontología* [Diagnosis and treatment of anxiety in the elderly, Major

Geriatric Disorders Series. *Protocols of the Spanish Society of Geriatrics and Gerontology*]. Available online at www.saludaliamedica.com/Med/protocolos/segg/ SEGG_ansiedad/protocolo.htm.

Perez-Franco B., Turabian-Fernandez J. L. (2006) Is the orthodox approach to depression in primary care valid?. *Aten. Primaria* **37**, 37–9.

Peveler R., Carson A., Rodin G. (2002) Depression in medical patients. *Br. Med. J.* **325**, 149–52.

Tellez-Lapeira J. M., Cerecedo-Perez M. J., Pascual-Pascual P., Buitrago-Ramirez F., Buitrago-Ramirez, F. (2005) Mental health on the threshold of the XXIst century: Primary care in the forefront – Are we up to the challenge? *Aten. Primaria* **35**, 61–3.

Tizón J. L. (1996) *Componentes Psicológicos de la Práctica Médica: Una Perspectiva desde la Atención Primaria* [Psychological Components of Medical Practice from the Primary Care Perspective], 4th edn. Barcelona: Doyma.

Von Korff M., Glasgow R. E., Sharpe M. (2002) Organizing care for chronic illness. *Br. Med. J.* **325**, 92–4.

United States of America

Professor Tom Campbell, Professor of Family Medicine, University of Rochester, NY, and Professor Jeffrey M. Lyness, Professor of Psychiatry, University of Rochester, NY

Health-care system

Miss LC's case is a typical presentation of an elderly depressed patient who comes to her primary care physician (PCP: either a family physician or internist in the USA) with somatic complaints (often pain) and minimizes or denies depressive symptoms. Our comments reflect general themes which are commonplace across the USA but must be tempered by recognition that the USA does not have a national health-care system. There are wide variations in practice due to factors including state and local government policies (even regarding local implementation of federal programs such as Medicare and Medicaid), private insurance companies, and other local 'cultural' practices of physicians.

Diagnosis

Miss LC's PCP is likely to accurately diagnose her with major depression 50–75% of the time, depending upon her presentation and how many other medical issues her PCP needs to address during the visit. A major barrier that PCPs face in diagnosing depression is lack of time and the 'competing demands' of each medical visit. Most elderly patients have three to four medical problems that must be addressed during a routine 15–30-minute visit, and these acute needs often compete with other important issues such as the recognition of depression.

Most PCPs diagnose major depression by clinical history, but rarely conduct a formal mental status examination or psychiatric interview and may only specifically ask a few of the nine diagnostic symptoms of major depression. An increasing number of PCPs are using the PHQ-9 (Patient Health Questionnaire) completed by the patient, for purposes of both making the diagnosis of depression and monitoring treatment. This questionnaire has become the predominant screening tool used by US PCPs, although probably the majority of practices do not use this or any other tool routinely. In the absence of evidence from the history (including review of systems) or examination suggesting new-onset or worsening physical disease as a potential contributor toward the depression, most PCPs probably would not order any laboratory tests as part of the initial work-up, although a few might order a thyroid function test or other screening blood work (e.g. complete blood count, serum electrolytes).

Management

Most cases of mild to moderate major depression in elderly patients are managed solely by PCPs. Referral to a psychiatrist occurs when the depression is severe or treatment refractory, there is concern about suicide risk, or there are other psychiatric co-morbidities. Most of these patients are treated with antidepressant medications, often selective serotonin reuptake inhibitors (SSRIs). In our region, she would most likely be offered escitalopram, citalopram or sertraline, although some PCPs would offer duloxetine as a first choice, given her coexisting pain and the recent marketing campaign for this medication for depression and pain. Even if offered antidepressants, many patients will refuse or not adhere to recommended treatment for a sufficient duration to adequately assess treatment response, and most PCPs will not see her back in the office quickly enough (e.g. within one to two weeks) to maximize adherence

Few such patients would be referred for psychotherapy due to multiple barriers including lack of access to psychotherapy especially for elderly patients, increased cost, and patient resistance to psychotherapy. Most PCPs would offer some degree of psycho-education, support and advice to increase socialization, possibly in conjunction with some degree of contact with the patient's family members. Again, there is great variability in how many of these services are offered and the skill with which they are administered.

Guidelines

There are many national and regional guidelines for the management of depression in primary care, and while they are widely accepted in principle, in practice they are often not followed. Many physicians are starting to use the principles of chronic disease management or Wagner's Chronic Care Model

(Wagner *et al.* 2001) to manage depression. These approaches include a multi-disciplinary approach with treatment protocols, intensive patient education and follow-up and use of patient registries. Three quality measures for the depression treatment have been widely accepted (including by HEDIS – Health plan Employer Data and Information Set, established by the National Committee for Quality Assurance) and are being tracked and reported by insurance companies. These include the optimal clinician contact and follow-up of patients diagnosed with depression and whether patients stay on their antidepressant medications both acutely and chronically. Some insurance companies are starting to use these and other quality measures to rate physicians' clinical care and adjust their financial compensation, an approach called 'Pay for Performance'. At the time of writing Medicare is about to begin such a program. It is expected, but yet to be demonstrated, that the inclusion of these depression quality measures in physician 'report cards' and pay-for-performance reimbursement systems will result in improvement in depression care.

Barriers to optimal care

In the present system there are multiple barriers to the delivery of optimal care, including inequitable access to primary care across regions and ethnic groups, often inadequate access to specialty mental health care, lack of incentives to spend the needed time with patients and families, and lack of funding to support alternative models, such as the on-site collaborative care models that have received ample empirical support in the scientific literature (see section on Management in Chapter 6 and Unützer *et al.* 2002).

Patient resources

As for patient literature, some PCPs would offer literature on depression provided to them, often by pharmaceutical companies or by local/regional insurance providers. There also are national-level resources available, regarding depression in later life, such as those provided by the Geriatric Mental Health Foundation at www.gmhfonline.org/gmhf/consumer/index.html (also discussed in Chapter 7).

National Committee for Quality Assurance *HEDIS (Health Plan Employer Data and Information Set)*. Available online at http: //web.ncqa.org
Unützer J., Katon W., Callahan C., *et al.* (2002) Collaborative care management of late-life depression in the primary care setting. *J. Am. Med. Assoc.* **288**, 2836–45.

Index

Abelskov, Kirsten 149–52
aetiology of depression in later life 3–5
alcohol problems *see* case 4.1 (Mrs Ruth M) 55
Alekxandrova, Maria 143–5
Allen, Harry 86–8
Ames, David 140–3
anticholinergic side effects, TCAs 26, 28–9
antidepressant treatment *see* pharmacotherapy
anxiety and depression 5–6
anxiety management 29
Apathy Evaluation Scale Inventory 120
assessment of patients, international
    comparisons 104–6
augmentation regimens 27–8
Australia
    commentary on case 6.1 (Miss Laura C) 140–3
    health-care system 140–3
Awata, Syuichi 158–60

Bălan, Monica 168–71
barriers to services/treatment for older patients
    133, 134
    cross-cultural comparisons 108–9
Beck Depression Inventory (BDI) 118
behavioural activation technique 29–30
Benoit, Michel 152–3
bipolar disorder, practice guidelines 127
blood tests, primary care evaluation 8–9
Bremmer, Marijke 161–5
Brief Assessment Schedule Depression Cards
    (BASDEC) 118
Bulgaria
    commentary on case 6.1 (Miss Laura C)
    143–5
    health-care system 143–5

Cabane, Florence 152–3
Campbell, Tom 175–7
Canada

commentary on case 6.1 (Miss Laura C)
    145–8
    health-care system 145–8
carers and families *see* case 4.3
    (Mr Le Lin P) 67
Caribbean Culture-Specific Screen (CCSS) for
    emotional distress 12–13, 116
case 3.1, request for sleeping tablets
    (Mr Seth Y) 33
case 3.1 commentaries
    editors' notes 51
    GP 33–6
    primary care nursing 36–9
case 3.2, loneliness and grief (Mrs Winifred E)
    39–40
case 3.2 commentaries
    editors' notes 51
    positive thoughts course 43–5
    primary care 40–3
case 3.3, panic attacks (Mrs Betty C) 45
case 3.3 commentaries
    consultant clinical psychologist 48–51
    editors' notes 52
    GP 45–8
case 4.1, hidden alcohol consumption (Mrs
    Ruth M) 55
case 4.1 commentaries
    editors' comments 79
    GP 55–60
    substance abuse counsellor 55–60
case 4.2, physical co-morbidity
    (Mr Wasif H) 60
case 4.2 commentaries
    consultant physician, medicine in the elderly
    63–7
    editors' comments 79–80
    GP 61–3
case 4.3, carers and families
    (Mr Le Lin P) 67

case 4.3 commentaries
  editors' comments 80
  GP 67–9
  social worker role 69–73
case 4.4, ethnically sensitive management (Mr
  Afzal C) 74
case 4.4 commentaries
  editors' comments 80
  GP 74–7
  voluntary sector organizations 77–8
case 5.1, depression with psychotic features
  (Mrs Paulette B) 83
case 5.1 commentaries
  editors' comments 99
  old-age psychiatrist 86–8
  primary care 83–5
case 5.2, risk of self-harm (Mrs Gladys H) 88–9
case 5.2 commentaries
  editors' comments 99
  GP 89–92
  old-age psychiatrist 92–3
case 5.3, depression and forgetfulness (Miss
  Lucy R) 93–4
case 5.3 commentaries
  editors' comments 100
  GP 94–6
  secondary care 96–9
case 6.1, breathlessness and irritability (Miss
  Laura C) 102
case 6.1, international commentaries 102–12
  assessment 104–6
  Australia 140–3
  barriers to treatment of older patients 108–9
  Bulgaria 143–5
  Canada 145–8
  Denmark 149–52
  France 152–3
  health-care systems 103–4
  Hong Kong 155–7
  Japan 158–60
  management 106–8
  Netherlands 161–5
  Norway 166–8
  presentation of depression 104
  protocols, guidelines and initiatives 109–12
  Romania 168–71
  Spain 171–4
  systems working together 108
  USA 175–7
Center for Epidemiological Studies Depression
  Scale (CES-D) 118

Challis, David 69–73
Cheshire, Mike 63–7
Chiu, Helen F. K. 155–7
Christensen, Kaj Sparle 149–52
citalopram 23
clinical evaluation of depression 8–9
clinical presentation of depression *see*
  presentation of depression in later life
Cocksedge, Simon 89–92
cognitive behavioural therapy (CBT) 18, 29
  guided self-help 20–2
collaborative care model of depression
  management 22–3
community-based group involvement, ethnic
  elders 13
concordance with treatment 17–18, 23–4
cross-cultural screening instruments 116

Danczak, Avril 61–3
dementia
  effects of pharmacotherapy for depression 24
  effects on presentation of depression 1–2,
    5–6
  screening tools 119, 120
Denmark
  commentary on case 6.1 (Miss Laura C) 149–52
  health-care system 149–52
depression treatment, practice guidelines
  120–7
diagnosis of depression in later life 5, 6, 7, 7
  clinical under-diagnosis 2–3
  core and additional symptoms 5, 6
  screening questions 7
Dicker, Alexandru 168–71
Dornan, Ceri 33–6
Dowrick, Christopher 40–3
drug interactions 27
DSM-IV criteria for depression 1, 5, 6
duloxetine 27

electroconvulsive therapy (ECT), indications
  for treatment 27–8
engaging the patient, ethnic elders 13 *see also*
  concordance with treatment
Engedal, Knut 166–8
epidemiology of depression in later life 1–3
  association with handicap 2
  clinical under-diagnosis 2–3
  criteria for depression 1
  effects of dementia 1–2
  effects of physical illness 1–2

epidemiology of depression in later life (cont.)
  effects of socio-economic status 2
  importance of early identification 2–3
  lack of assessment, diagnosis and
      management 2–3
  potential risk factors 2
  prevalence and incidence rates 1–2
  profile of high-risk groups 2–3
  range and fluctuation of symptom severity 2
  range of symptom presentation 2
  targeted screening programmes 2–3
escitalopram 23
ethnic elders
  ageing of immigrant population 9
  barriers to services 133, 134
  migration to the UK 9
ethnic elders and depression 9–13
  age-related factors 10
  assessment considerations 11, 12
  barriers to services 133, 134
  beliefs about depression 10, 11
  Caribbean Culture-Specific Screen (CCSS)
      for emotional distress 12–13, 116
  community-based group involvement 13
  course of depression 11
  cross-cultural screening instruments 12–13,
      116
  culturally sensitive assessment 11, 12
  culture-specific descriptions of distress 11
  effective communication 11, 12
  engaging the patient 13
  ethnically sensitive management see case 4.4
      (Mr Afzal C) 74
  faith-based group involvement 13
  interpreters 12
  level of risk 9
  management issues 13
  misconceptions about depression 10, 11
  multiple jeopardy concept 9
  pharmacological interventions 13
  prevalence of chronic medical conditions 10
  prevalence of depression 9–10
  psychological interventions 13
  psychosocial issues 10
  reluctance to use psychiatric services 10
  reluctance to use secondary mental health
      services 10
  risk factors 10
  screening scales for ethnic elders 12–13
  symptoms of depression 11
  translators 12
  utilization of GP services 10
  working with the family 13
ethnic minorities in the UK
  history of UK immigration 9
  population age structure 9
  prevalence of depression 9–10
  prevalence of self-harm and suicide 9–10
ethnically sensitive management see case 4.4
    (Mr Afzal C) 74
exercise and activity, to avoid or counter
    depression 29–30

faith-based group involvement, ethnic elders
    13 see also voluntary sector organizations
family
  involvement with ethnic elders 13
  work with 30, 67
  see also case 4.3
    (Mr Le Lin P) 67
Ferreiro Guri, José Antonio 171–4
fluoxetine 26–7
Flynn, Eleanor 140–3
forgetfulness and depression see case 5.3 (Miss
    Lucy R) 93–4
Fox, Chris 96–9
France
  commentary on case 6.1 (Miss Laura C)
    152–3
  health-care system 152–3

General Medical Services Contract (GMS),
    Quality and Outcomes Framework
    (QuOF) 7, 7
Geriatric Depression Scale (GDS) 7, 114–16
  cross-cultural application 116
  use for ethnic elders 12–13
Geriatric Mental State Examination, criteria for
    depression 1
guided self-help (GSH) 20–1
  implementation 21–2
guidelines see practice guidelines

Hamilton Rating Scale for Depression
    (HAM-D) 120, 123
handicap
  and risk of depression 2
  definition 2
  link with depression 30
  social interventions 30
health-care systems, international comparisons
    103–4

Hong Kong
    commentary on case 6.1 (Miss Laura C) 155–7
    health care system 155–7
Honma, Akira 158–60
Hughes, Jane 69–73
hypochondriasis 5–6

ICD-10 criteria for depression 5, 6
Iliffe, Steve 94–6
immigrant elderly population *see* ethnic elders
international commentaries on depression
        management 102–12
    assessment 104–6
    Australia 140–3
    barriers to treatment of older patients 108–9
    Bulgaria 143–5
    Canada 145–8
    case 6.1 (Miss Laura C) 102
    Denmark 149–52
    France 152–3
    health-care systems 103–4
    Hong Kong 155–7
    Japan 158–60
    management 106–8
    Netherlands 161–5
    Norway 166–8
    presentation of depression 104
    protocols, guidelines and initiatives 109–12
    Romania 168–71
    Spain 171–4
    systems working together 108
    USA 175–7
inter-personal psychotherapy (IPT) 29

Japan
    commentary on case 6.1 (Miss Laura C)
        158–60
    health-care system 158–60

Katona, Cornelius 96–9

Lambat, Ahmed I. 77–8
legal framework 134, 135
Lester, Helen 83–5
Li, D. K. T. 155–7
Licht-Strunk, Els 161–5
literature and online resources for patients 127–31
lofepramine 26–7
loneliness and grief *see* case 3.2 (Mrs Winifred
        E) 39–40
Lyness, Jeffrey M. 175–7

major depression 5–6
management of depression
    cognitive behavioural therapy (CBT) 18,
        20–2
    collaborative care model 22–3
    concordance with treatment 17–18, 23
    effective treatments 17
    general principles of treatment 17–23
    goals of treatment 17–18
    guided self-help 20–2
    international comparisons 106–8
    pharmacotherapy 23–9
    polypharmacy 17–18
    primary care setting 17
    psychological interventions 27–8,
        29–30
    self-help 20–2
    self-medication 17–18
    social interventions 30
    stepped care model 18–22
    use of St John's wort 17–18
Martin, Sue 43–5
Mateos, Raimundo 171–4
medical services for late-life
        depression 133
memory disturbance 5–6
mental capacity 134, 135
Mental Capacity Act 2005,
        England 134, 135
Mental Health Act 1983,
        England 134
mental health law 134
mental state assessment, primary care
        evaluation 8–9 *see also case studies*
Mini-Mental Status Examination
        (MMSE) 119
mirtazepine 23, 27
moclobemide 27
Montgomery Äsberg Depression Rating Scale
        (MADRAS) 120, 126
Morley, Michael 48–51
Murray, Elizabeth 55–60

Netherlands
    commentary on case 6.1 (Miss Laura C)
        161–5
    health-care system 161–5
Norway
    commentary on case 6.1 (Miss Laura C)
        166–8
    health-care system 166–8

Oliver, James 55–60
online resources for patients 127–31
Orientation–Memory–Concentration (OMC)
    test 119, 120

pain, and risk of depression 2
panic attacks *see* case 3.3 (Mrs Betty C) 45
parkinsonism 28–9
paroxetine 27, 28–9
patient engagement in treatment 23–4 *see also*
    concordance with treatment
Patient Health Questionnaire (PHQ)
    diagnostic tool 116, 117
    measurement of severity 116, 118, 120
    screening tool 116, 117
patient history, primary care evaluation 8–9
patient information
    education material 127–31
    literature and online resources 127–31
    self-help material and groups 131–2
pharmacotherapy 23–9
    augmentation regimens 27–8
    choice of antidepressant 23
    citalopram 23
    combination with psychological
        interventions 29
    concordance with treatment 17–18, 23–4
    discontinuation symptoms 27
    dosages 26, 27
    drug interactions 27
    duloxetine 27
    effects on dementia 24
    efficacy 24–5, 26
    epilepsy caution 27
    escitalopram 23
    ethnic elders 13
    fluoxetine 26–7
    gastrointestinal haemorrhage caution 27
    implications of placebo response 24
    indications for psychiatric referral 27–8, 28
    initiating antidepressant treatment 23–4
    inter-individual variations in older people 28–9
    lofepramine 26–7
    mirtazepine 23, 27
    moclobemide 27
    'non-specific' factors in recovery 24
    paroxetine 27, 28–9
    patient and carer views on antidepressants 23
    patient engagement in treatment 23–4
    patients who do not respond 27–8, 28
    polypharmacy 17–18

self-medication 17–18
sertraline 23
side effects 26–7, 28–9
sources of response variability 28–9
speed of response in older people 27
SSRIs 26–7, 28–9
St John's wort 17–18
tricyclic antidepressants (TCAs) 23, 26, 27,
    28–9
venlafaxine 27
physical examination, primary care evaluation
    8–9
physical illness, and depression 1–2, 60 *see also*
    case 4.2 (Mr Wasif H)
placebo response 24
polypharmacy 17–18
positive thoughts course 43–5
practice guidelines
    bipolar disorder 127
    treatment of depression 120–7
precipitating factors for depression in later life
    3–5
presentation of depression in later life 5–9
    anxiety 5–6
    clinical evaluation 8–9
    clinical presentation 5–6
    core and additional symptoms 5, 6
    cross-cultural comparisons 104
    diagnosis 5, 6, 7, 7
    DSM-IV criteria 5, 6
    effects of dementia 5–6
    hypochondriasis 5–6
    ICD-10 criteria 5, 6
    major depression 5–6
    memory disturbance 5–6
    primary care evaluation 8–9
    rating scales 8
    see also ethnic elders
prevalence of depression, ethnic minorities in
    the UK 9–10
primary care evaluation of depression 8–9
    see also case histories
problem-solving treatment (PST) 29
protective factors for depression in later life 3–4
Protheroe, Jo 67–9
protocols and pathways for depression
    management 135, 136
protocols, guidelines and initiatives,
    international comparisons 109–12
psychiatric referral, antidepressant-resistant
    depression 27–8, 28

psychodynamic psychotherapy 29
psychological interventions 27–8, 29–30
    anxiety management 29
    behavioural activation 29–30
    cognitive behavioural therapy (CBT) 29
    combination with pharmacotherapy 29
    ethnic elders 13
    exercise and activity 29–30
    family work 30
    inter-personal psychotherapy (IPT) 29
    problem-solving treatment (PST) 29
    psychodynamic psychotherapy 29
psychotherapy, augmentation regimens 27–8
psychotic features with depression
    see case 5.1 (Mrs Paulette B) 83
Pusey, Helen 36–9

Quality and Outcomes Framework (QuOF) of
    the General Medical Services Contract
    (GMS) 7, 7

Rait, Greta 74–7
Ratcliffe, Joy 92–3
rating scales, use in evaluation of depression 8
religious organisations 133 see also faith-based
    group involvement; voluntary sector
    organizations
residential care, rates of depression 1–2
resources
    Apathy Evaluation Scale Inventory 120
    assessment of severity 118, 120, 123, 126
    Beck Depression Inventory 118
    bipolar disorder practice guidelines 127
    Brief Assessment Schedule Depression Cards
        (BASDEC) 118
    Caribbean Culture-Specific Screen (CCSS)
        for emotional distress 116
    Center for Epidemiological Studies
        Depression Scale (CES-D) 118
    cross-cultural screening instruments 116
    Geriatric Depression Scale (GDS)
        114–16
    Hamilton Rating Scale for Depression
        (HAM-D) 120, 123
    legal framework 134, 135
    literature and online resources for patients
        127–31
    mental capacity 134, 135
    mental health law 134
    Mini-Mental Status Examination
        (MMSE) 119

Montgomery Äsberg Depression Rating
    Scale (MADRAS) 120, 126
Orientation–Memory–Concentration
    (OMC) test 119, 120
patient education material 127–31
Patient Health Questionnaire (PHQ) 116,
    117, 118, 120
protocols and pathways 135, 136
screening for dementia 119, 120
screening for depression in older people
    114–19, 120
SelfCARE(D) 118
self-help material and groups 131–2
services for older people with depression
    132–3, 134
suicide risk assessment and suicide
    prevention 118
treatment of depression practice guidelines
    120–7
World Health Organization Well-Being
    Index (WHO-5) 118, 119
risk assessment, suicidality 8–9
risk factors for depression in later life 2, 3–5
    profile of high risk groups 2–3
Robert, Philippe H. 152–3
Romania
    commentary on case 6.1 (Miss Laura C)
        168–71
    health-care system 168–71
Ruault, Geneviève 152–3

Sanaker, Harald 166–8
screening for dementia 119, 120
screening programmes for depression in later
    life 2–3
screening questions for depression in later life,
    7
screening scales for ethnic elders 12–13
screening tools for depression in older people
    114–19, 120
selective serotonin reuptake inhibitors (SSRIs)
    26–7, 28–9
SelfCARE(D) 118
self-harm 8–9
    among ethnic minority adults 9–10see also
        suicide risk assessment
self-help interventions for depression 20–2
self-help material and groups 131–2
self-medication 17–18
self-neglect 8–9
sertraline 23

services for older people with depression
132–3, 134
barriers to services 133, 134
medical services 133
religious organizations 133
social care 133
voluntary services 133
severity assessment, Patient Health
Questionnaire (PHQ) 116, 118, 120
Shulman, Kenneth 145–8
sleeping tablets request *see* case 3.1
(Mr Seth Y) 33
social care services for late-life depression 133
social interventions 30
addressing sources of handicap 30
social isolation, and risk of depression 2, 30
socio-economic status, and risk of depression
in later life 2
Spain
commentary on case 6.1 (Miss Laura C)
171–4
health care system 171–4
specialist services, international comparisons 108
SPICE heuristic 95
St John's wort 17–18
stepped care model of depression management
18–22
guided self-help 20–2
practical considerations 22
self-help 20–2

Stoychev, Kaloyan 143–5
substance abuse *see* case 4.1 (Mrs Ruth M) 55
suicide, among ethnic minority adults 9–10
suicide prevention resources 118
suicide risk assessment
primary care evaluation 8–9
resources 88–9, 118*see also* case 5.2 (Mrs
Gladys H) 88–9
syndrome of inappropriate antidiuretic
hormone secretion (SIADH) 28–9

Tătaru, Nicoleta 168–71
Thompson, Ruth 45–8
treatment-emergent parkinsonism 28–9
tricyclic antidepressants (TCAs) 23
drug interactions 27
side effects 26, 28–9

Upshur, Ross 145–8
USA
commentary on case 6.1 (Miss Laura C)
175–7
health-care system 175–7

validated tools, use for diagnosis of depression 7
venlafaxine 27
voluntary sector organizations 77–8, 133

World Health Organization Well-Being Index
(WHO-5) 118, 119